Mosby's 1997 AssessTest

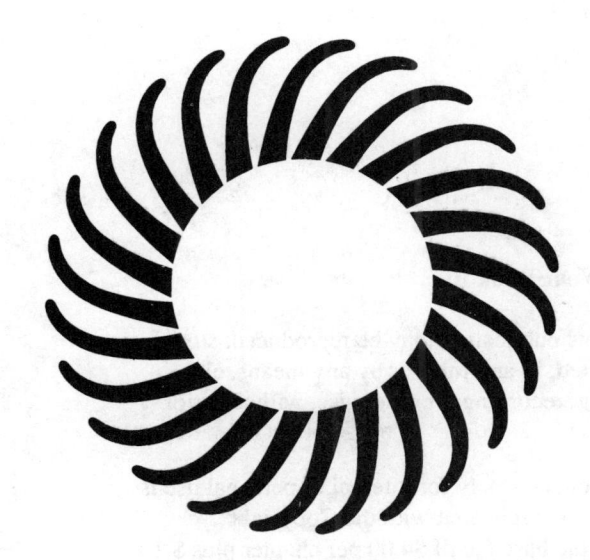

A practice exam for RN licensure

SAXTON ♦ PELIKAN ♦ NEEDLEMAN ♦ NUGENT

Mosby

St. Louis Baltimore Boston Carlsbad Chicago Naples New York Philadelphia Portland
London Madrid Mexico City Singapore Sydney Tokyo Toronto Wiesbaden

Mosby
Dedicated to Publishing Excellence

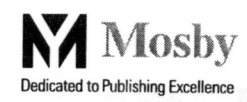

A Times Mirror
Company

Vice President and Publisher: Nancy L. Coon
Senior Editor: Susan R. Epstein
Senior Developmental Editor: Beverly J. Copland
Manufacturing Supervisor: Theresa Fuchs
Senior Composition Specialist: Chris Robinson

Copyright © 1997 by Mosby–Year Book, Inc.

All rights reserved. No part of this publication may be reproduced, stored in a retrieval system, or transmitted, in any form or by any means, electronic, mechanical, photocopying, recording, or otherwise, without prior written permission of the publisher.

Permission to photocopy or reproduce solely for internal or personal use is permitted for libraries or other users registered with the Copyright Clearance Center, provided that the base fee of $4.00 per chapter plus $.10 per page is paid directly to the Copyright Clearance Center, 27 Congress Street, Salem, MA 01970. This consent does not extend to other kinds of copying, such as copying for general distribution, for advertising or promotional purposes, for creating new collected works, or for resale.

Printed in the United States of America
Composition by Mosby Electronic Publishing
Printing/binding by Plus Communications

Mosby–Year Book, Inc.
11830 Westline Industrial Drive
St. Louis, Missouri 63146

International Standard Book Number 0-8151-8507-3

97 98 / 9 8 7 6 5 4 3 2 1

Editorial Panel

Editor

Dolores F. Saxton, R.N., B.S. in Ed., M.A., M.P.S, Ed.D.

Private Practice,
President, D.F.S. Enterprises, Ltd.
Farmingdale, New York

Associate Editors

Phyllis K. Pelikan, R.N., A.A.S., B.S., M.A.

Professor Emeritus,
Nassau Community College
Garden City, New York
President, P.K.P. Books, Inc.
Wantagh, New York

Selma R. Needleman, R.N., B.A., M.A.

Professor Emeritus,
Nassau Community College
Garden City, New York
Adjunct Nursing Faculty,
St. Petersburg Junior College
St. Petersburg, Florida

Patricia M. Nugent, R.N., A.A.S., B.S., M.S., Ed.M., Ed.D.

Associate Professor of Nursing,
Nassau Community College
Garden City, New York

Content Editors

Phyllis Portnoy Cohen, R.N., R.N.C., M.S.

Perinatal Clinical Nurse Specialist
Long Island Jewish Medical Center
Division of OB/GYN
New Hyde Park, New York

JoAnn Schmidt Festa, R.N.C., A.A.S, B.S., M.S., Ph.D.

Professor of Nursing
Nassau Community College
Garden City, New York

Colleen Glavinspiehs, R.N.C, B.S., M.S.N., D.N.Sc., F.N.P.

Associate Professor of Nursing
Burlington County Community College
Burlington, New Jersey

Christina Algiere Kasprisin, R.N., M.S., M.S.

Lecturer in Nursing
University of Vermont School of Nursing
Burlington, Vermont

Anita Throwe, R.N., B.S.N., M.S.

Associate Professor of Nursing
Medical University of South Carolina, College
 of Nursing
Program at Francis Marion University
Florence, South Carolina

Statistical Consultant

Terry O'Dwyer, B.S., Ph.D.

Professor of Physics
Nassau Community College
Garden City, New York

Contributors

Janet T. Ihlenfeld, R.N., B.S.N., M.S.N., Ph.D.

D'Youville College
Buffalo, New York

Bruce A. Scott, R.N., B.S.N., M.S.N.

Mount Saint Mary's College
Los Angeles, California

Anita Throwe, R.N., B.S.N., M.S.

Medical University of South Carolina, College
    of Nursing
Florence, South Carolina

Patricia E. Zander, R.N., B.S.N., M.S.N.

Viterbo College
LaCrosse, Wisconsin

Mary Crosley, R.N., B.S., M.S.

Suffolk County Community College
Brentwood, New York

John Harper, R.N., M.S.N.

Neuman College
Aston, Pennslyvania

Ayda G. Nambayan, R.N., O.C.N., B.S.N., M.Ed.

University of Alabama at Birmingham School
    of Nursing
Birmingham, Alabama

Ruth Gouner, R.N., M.S.

Nicholls State University
Thibodaux, Louisiana

Shirley Ann Dufresne, R.N., B.S., M.S.N.

University of Massachusetts
North Dartmouth, Massachusetts

JoAnn Schmidt Festa, R.N.C., A.A.S., B.S., M.S., Ph.D.

Nassau Community College
Garden City, New York

Ellen M. Chiocca, R.N., R.N.C., B.S.N., M.S.N.

Loyola University, Marcella Niehoff School of Nursing
Chicago, Illinois

Carol Flaugher, R.N., B.S.N., M.S.

State University of New York at Buffalo School
    of Nursing
Buffalo, New York

Barbara Fomenko Harrah, R.N., B.S. Ed., M.S.N.

The Ohio Valley Hospital School of Nursing
Steubenville, Ohio

Laurie A. Gasperi Kaudewitz, R.N., R.N.C., B.S.N., M.S.N.

East Tennessee State University School of Nursing
Johnson City, Tennessee

Cecilia Mukai, R.N., B.S., M.S.N.

University of Hawaii at Hilo
Hilo, Hawaii

Doris E. Nicholas, R.N., B.S., M.S., Ph.D.

Howard University College of Nursing
Washington, District of Columbia

Linda Carman Copel, R.N., B.S.N., M.S., M.S.N., Ph.D.

Villanova University College of Nursing
Villanova, Pennsylvania

Susan V. Gille, R.N., B.S.N., M.S.N., M.S.P.H., Ph.D.

Missouri Western State College
St. Joseph, Missouri

Dorothy B. Lary, R.N., C.S., B.S.N., M.S.N.

Louisiana College
Pineville, Louisiana

Sheila Elizabeth Miller, R.N., B.S.N., M.S.N.

Auburn University, School of Nursing
Auburn University, Alabama

Marsha Dowell, R.N., B.S.N., M.S.N.

University of Virginia, School of Nursing
Charlottesville, Virginia

Leann Eaton, R.N., B.S.N., M.S.N.

Jewish Hospital School of Nursing
St Louis, Missouri

Jane Flickinger, R.N., B.S., M.S.N.

Rochester Community College
Rochester, Minnesota

Christina Algiere Kasprisin, R.N., M.S., M.S.

University of Vermont School of Nursing
Burlington, Vermont

Melodie Olson, R.N., B.S.N., M.S.N., Ph.D.

San Antonio College
San Antonio, Texas

Linda Owen Rimer, R.N., B.S.N., M.S.E.

University of Arkansas at Little Rock
Little Rock, Arkansas

Lynn Wolfe Andrews, R.N., A.S., B.S.N., M.S.N.

St. Mary's Hospital School of Nursing
Huntington, West Virginia

Michael Dreyer, R.N., B.S.N., M.N.

LaSalle University, School of Nursing
Philadelphia, Pennsylvania

Mary Reuther Herring, R.N., B.S.N., M.S.N.

Motorola Incorporated and University of Phoenix
Phoenix, Arizonia

Bernadette Kahler, R.N., B.S.N., M.N.

Kansas Newman College
Wichita, Kansas

Joanne Lavin, R.N., B.S.N., M.S., M.Ed., Ed.D.

Kingsborough Community College
Brooklyn, New York

Pamela M. Lemmon, R.N., B.S.N., M.S.N.

Gannon University
Youngstown, Ohio

Diane Melancon, R.N., A.D.N., B.S.N., M.S.N., Ed.D.

San Antonio College
San Antonio, Texas

Jeanne M. Millett, R.N., F.N.P., B.S., M.S., Ed.D.

Albany Medical Center Hospital Lifestar Regional Trauma System
Albany, New York

Ann T. Muller, R.N., B.S., M.Ed., Ph.D.

Private Practice
Dallas, Texas

Mary Ann S. Rogers, R.N., A.D.N., B.S.N., M.S.N., Ed.D.

University of South Carolina at Aiken
Aiken, South Carolina

Ann D. Sprengel, R.N., B.S.N., M.S.N.

Southeast Missouri State University
Cape Girardeau, Missouri

Janet R. Weber, R.N., B.S.N., M.S.N.

Southeast Missouri State University
Cape Girardeau, Missouri

Mary H. West, R.N., C.C.N., M.S.

Bob Jones University
Greenville, South Carolina

Judy E. White, R.N., B.S.N, M.A., M.S.N.

Rockland Community College
Suffern, New York

Carolyn Browne, R.N., M.A.

Olsten Kimberly QualityCare
Westbury, New York

H. Carolyn Carpenter, R.N., B.A., M.S.N.

Presbyterian Hospital School of Nursing
Charlotte, North Carolina

Penelope L. Daniels, R.N., C.S., A.D.N.S., B.S., B.S.N., M.S.

St. Mary's Hospital School of Nursing
Huntington, West Virginia

Teresa Marie Dobrzykowski, R.N., A.S.N., B.S.N., M.S.N.

Indiana University at South Bend
South Bend, Indiana

Su Lin Durrwachter, R.N., B.S.N., M.S.N.

Baton Rouge General Medical Center School of Nursing
Baton Rouge, Louisiana

Carmel A. Esposito, R.N., B.S.N., M.S.N., Ed.D.

Ohio Valley Hospital School of Nursing
Steubenville, Ohio

Margaret Comerford Freda, R.N., B.S., B.S.N., M.A., Ed.D.

Albert Einstein College of Medicine
Bronx, New York

Caroline H. Hollshwandner, R.N., B.S.N., M.A., Ph.D.

Allentown College of St. Francis de Sales
Center Valley, Pennslyvania

Carole J. Labby, R.N., B.S.N., M.S.

College of the Mainland
Houston, Texas

Barbara C. Martin, R.N., C.S., B.S.N., M.S.

University of Tulsa
Tulsa, Oklahoma

Marilyn M. Mohr, R.N., B.S.N., M.S.N.

Missouri Baptist Medical Center School of Nursing
St. Louis, Missouri

Patricia O'Neill, R.N., M.S.

State University of New York at Stony Brook, School of Nursing
Stony Brook, New York

Lois H. Rafenski, R.N., A.A.S., B.S., M.Ed., Ed.D.

State University of New York at Farmingdale
Farmingdale, New York

Christina M. Swieton, R.N., B.S.N., M.S.

California Medical Research
La Mesa, California

Ruth B. Taylor, R.N., M.S.N., M.Ed.

La Mar University, College of Health and Behavioral Sciences
Beaumont, Texas

Cecilia M. Tiller, R.N., B.S.N., M.N., D.S.N.

Medical College of Georgia School of Nursing
Augusta, Georgia

Deborah Williams, R.N., A.S., B.A., M.S.N.

Western Kentucky University
Bowling Green, Kentucky

Frances A. Wollner, R.N., B.S., B.S.N., M.N.

Grand Island, New York

Preface

For almost 15 years MOSBY'S *AssessTest* has been helping students prepare for licensure. The National Council Licensure Examination for Registered Nurses (NCLEX-RN) in the United States and the Nurse Registration-Licensure Examination in Canada are based on normally encountered nursing situations that cross clinical disciplines. Mosby's *AssessTest* has been designed to assist nursing students to prepare for these examinations by evaluating their level of knowledge and providing feedback on clinical areas that may need further study. With the change in the NCLEX-RN to computerized adaptive testing (CAT), faculty and students need the benefits offered by the *AssessTest* now more than ever. These benefits provide both institutional and individual feedback that evaluates students' comprehension and assists faculty to evaluate specific curriculum content.

The 1996 *AssessTest* reflects the new NCLEX-CAT Examination. Approximately two-thirds of the students taking the NCLEX-RN pass or fail after 75 questions, the minimum number of questions every candidate must complete. *AssessTest*, therefore, includes four content-integrated tests of 75 questions each. Dividing the 300 questions into these four tests gives students a feel for the scope of content that will be covered on the NCLEX. It also allows faculty to administer each of the tests comfortably in a 90-minute block of time.

Like the NCLEX-RN, the multiple-choice questions in *AssessTest* offer four possible answers, and each question is independent of any other question. Each of the four tests covers nursing content equally in the core clinical areas of medicine, surgery, pediatrics, mental health, and childbearing and women's health. The test plan for *AssessTest* adheres to the guidelines for the components of Client Needs and Phases of the Nursing Process published by the National Council of State Boards of Nursing, Inc. in *NCLEX-RN Test Plan for the National Council Licensure Examination for Registered Nurses—Effective Date: October 1995*.

All 300 questions in *AssessTest* have been field tested by graduating students representing a broad geographic distribution and enrolled in baccalaureate, associate degree, and diploma nursing programs. This field testing ensures quality and validity of the questions. The questions reflect the latest knowledge, activities, procedures, medications, nursing diagnoses, and terminology encountered by the entry level nurse.

AssessTest provides each student with a computerized performance evaluation that includes:

- an overall summary of test results with comparison to the norm group, indicating how student ranks compared to peers nationwide,
- a personal profile indicating clinical areas of greatest need for further study to help student plan study time more effectively,
- a summary comparing performance to the norm group in nursing process, cognitive level, client needs, and clinical area that assists in determining strengths and weaknesses, and
- a list of questions answered incorrectly and the response selected so the student can refer back to the test and review mistakes.

Each student also receives a booklet containing answers and rationales for every question on the test, which promotes further learning and understanding by explaining why the correct option was correct and why the other three were not correct. MOSBY'S *AssessTest* is a valuable diagnostic tool that provides extensive feedback on performance and makes even incorrect selections a learning opportunity.

The institutional profile is available to schools with 10 or more participants and is provided when answer sheets for the entire group are submitted for processing in a single batch. The extensive institutional analysis assists faculty in preparing their students for the exam and in evaluating the school's curriculum. The evaluative feedback for an institution:

- summarizes and compares group's scores to the RN norm group and program-specific norm group so faculty can determine how students rank among peers,
- graphically summarizes performance overall and in nursing process, cognitive level, clinical area, and client needs, which helps identify strengths and weaknesses of curriculum,
- provides summary of group performance compared to both norm groups to assist faculty in curriculum evaluation,

- analyzes group's performance by clinical areas for nursing process, cognitive level, and client needs, which assists faculty in determining strengths and weaknesses of curriculum,
- includes percentage of students choosing the correct answer for each question, which assists faculty in identifying specific questions their students found difficult,
- includes a student roster indicating the percent correct and percentile ranking relative to the RN norm group, assisting faculty in identifying students who need special help, and
- provides faculty a comparison of scores with last year's test that enables them to evaluate consistency of student performance and curriculum.

It is readily apparent that the extensive analysis, statistics, and comparisons offered by MOSBY'S *AssessTest* can best be achieved using a standardized test. The nursing content that is tested and the structure of the questions all parallel the NCLEX-RN, providing a highly effective evaluation of students' readiness for the examination.

We would like to thank the following persons who have contributed their time and talents: Susan Epstein, our Acquisitions Editor, for her invaluable assistance and friendship; Beverly Copland, our Senior Developmental Editor, for her management of our project; Barbara Moore for her coordination of field testing; Edith Augustson and Mary Vella for their diligence in the preparation of our manuscript; our contributors and consultants; the students who participated in the field testing ventures; the proctors who administered the field tests; and our families for their support and sacrifice.

We sincerely hope that the *AssessTest* experience is challenging and beneficial to you. Good luck!

THE EDITORS

Contents

Introduction

What is *AssessTest*, 10
Categories of Abilities Measured by *AssessTest*, 10
How to Maximize the Benefits of Your *AssessTest* Experience, 11
Computer Evaluation, 15

AssessTest

Directions for Taking *AssessTest*, 16
Directions for Group Administration of *AssessTest*, 18
Cover Sheet for Group-Administered *AssessTest*, 19
Comprehensive Examination 1, 21
Comprehensive Examination 2, 31
Comprehensive Examination 3, 41
Comprehensive Examination 4, 51

Appendices

   A State and Territorial Boards of Nursing, 61
   B Canadian Provincial Registered Nurses Associations, 65

Introduction

WHAT IS AssessTest?

AssessTest is a computer-scored, multiple-choice examination designed to test essential nursing knowledge and evaluate ability to apply that knowledge to various clinical situations. The extensive computer analysis of your performance, which is the most outstanding feature of this test, will help you design effective and efficient plans for further study and review. Identification of your own specific strengths and weaknesses ought to eliminate much of the anxiety connected with deciding what material to study by giving you a sense of direction and a means of setting priorities. Designed to reflect the broad scope of basic nursing knowledge, *AssessTest* can be used for preparation and review in a variety of situations such as preparing for licensure examination, general evaluation for practicing nurses, review for nurses returning to work after an absence, or foreign-student preparation for qualifying examinations.

AssessTest consists of 4 randomly selected, content-integrated tests totaling 300 questions. Organized in a nursing process framework, the questions are constructed to reflect nursing situations that cross clinical disciplines. Clients rarely present an isolated health problem, and the nurse must be able to respond to individual needs regardless of the clinical area or diagnosis. The test requires you to respond to common human needs as well as to specific needs associated with given health problems.

CATEGORIES OF ABILITIES MEASURED BY *AssessTest*

Every question on *AssessTest* has been classified in each of five categories of abilities: (1) nursing behavior (phase of the nursing process), (2) cognitive level, (3) clinical area, (4) client needs, and (5) category of concern.

Because *AssessTest* is an evaluative study tool, we have included nursing content to equally represent the clinical areas of medicine, surgery, pediatrics, mental health, and childbearing and women's health. This approach should be recognized as a deliberate variation from the NCLEX-RN. However, to reflect the types of questions the student will have to answer on the national examination in the categories of Nursing Process and Client Needs, we have selected questions that reflect the percentages allocated to them in the NCLEX-RN Test Plan (October 1995). The questions used were randomly placed on the test after being selected from the pool of questions developed from the nationwide field testing. They reflect the latest activities, procedures, drugs, and nursing diagnoses.

Nursing behavior (phase of the nursing process)

In the United States and Canada, the licensure examinations are constructed in a nursing process framework. *AssessTest* also evaluates your ability to carry out the five components of the nursing process. These five components represent the various types of nursing behavior:

Assessment. The assessment phase of the nursing process involves gathering subjective and objective data about the client's health status from meaningful sources, grouping the data into categories, and communicating the information to others. The data base for making nursing decisions is determined through the assessing phase.

Analysis. In the analysis phase of the nursing process, the nurse interprets the data obtained during the assessment phase to identify the client's actual or potential health care needs and to formulate nursing diagnoses.

Planning. During the planning phase of the nursing process, the nurse designs strategies to correct, minimize, or prevent problems identified during the assessment and analysis phase; sets priorities for the problems diagnosed; develops both short-term and long-term goals with the client and/or client's family; establishes outcome criteria for nursing interventions; and writes the nursing care plan.

Implementation. In the implementation phase, the nurse initiates and completes the plan of care. The nurse may perform the care or assist, teach, counsel, or supervise the client, client's significant others, or other health team members to perform specific interventions based on the client's identified needs, diagnoses, priorities, and goals.

Evaluation. Through the evaluation component of the nursing process, the nurse determines the effectiveness of nursing intervention. In doing so, the nurse compares the actual outcomes with the expected outcomes to determine client compliance with and response to the intervention or therapy. The nurse uses the evaluation phase to identify whether the health care need still exists, which would require modification of the plan, or whether new health care needs have developed, which would require new interventions.

Cognitive level

In all nursing situations, real and hypothetical, various types of intellectual processes or cognitive abilities come into play. Four levels of cognitive ability are evaluated by *AssessTest*:

Knowledge. The knowledge level of the intellectual process requires recall of facts about principles, concepts, theories, terms, or procedures. Representing the most basic kind of mastery over subject matter, knowledge questions require the test taker to define, identify, or select.

Comprehension. The comprehension level presupposes the ability to recall knowledge and further requires an understanding or interpretation of the subject. Questions that require the test taker to interpret, explain, distinguish, or predict test intellectual ability to comprehend information.

Application. Building on the knowledge and comprehension levels, the application level requires the use of comprehended information in new situations. Questions that require the test taker to show, solve, modify, change, manipulate, use, demonstrate, or teach test intellectual ability to apply knowledge.

Analysis. Analysis assumes abilities in all three cognitive levels just discussed. This level requires the recognition of inherent structure and relationships between component parts. Questions that require the nurse to evaluate, differentiate, or interpret data from a variety of sources test analytic ability.

Clinical area

Each question has been coded as primarily pertaining to one of five clinical areas: **medical nursing, surgical nursing, childbearing and women's health nursing, pediatric nursing, or mental health nursing.**

Client needs

Client needs are those health care needs of the client which the nurse must address. The *AssessTest* evaluates four areas of client needs:

Support and promotion of physiologic and anatomic equilibrium. Meeting this need includes reducing risks that interfere with physiologic or anatomic integrity; promoting comfort and mobility; and providing basic care to assist, modify, or limit physiologic and anatomic adaptations.

An environment that is safe and conducive to effective therapeutic care. Addressing this need includes providing quality, goal-directed care that is coordinated, safe, and effective.

Education and other forms of health promotion to prevent, minimize, or correct actual or potential health problems. Fulfilling this need involves supporting optimal growth and development to provide for the achievement of the highest level of functioning. This level includes encouraging the use of support systems and self-care directed toward promoting the prevention, recognition, and treatment of disease throughout the life cycle.

Support and promotion of psychosocial and emotional equilibrium. Satisfying this need includes supporting individual emotional coping and adapting mechanisms to promote optimal emotional health while limiting or modifying those responses to crises which produce psychopathologic consequences.

Categories of concern

The categories of concern are indicators of the specific content areas within the broad clinical areas.

The following categories of concern are used in **medical, surgical, and pediatric nursing**: blood and immunity, cardiovascular, drug-related responses, growth and development, emotional needs related to health problems, fluid and electrolyte, endocrine, gastrointestinal, integumentary, neuromuscular, reproductive and genitourinary, respiratory, and skeletal.

The following categories of concern are used in **childbearing and women's health nursing**: drug-related responses, emotional needs related to childbearing and women's health, healthy childbearing, high-risk maternal-fetal conditions affecting childbearing, high-risk neonate, normal neonate, reproductive choices, reproductive problems, and women's health.

The following categories of concern are used in **mental health nursing**: anxiety, somatoform, and dissociative disorders; crisis situations; dementia, delirium, and other cognitive disorders; disorders first evident before adulthood; disorders of mood; disorders of personality; drug-related responses; eating disorders; emotional problems related to physical health and childbearing; personality development; schizophrenic disorders; substance abuse; and therapeutic relationships.

HOW TO MAXIMIZE THE BENEFITS OF YOUR *AssessTest* EXPERIENCE

Use this opportunity to become "test wise."

Do you really know what a multiple-choice question is? Do you know how to read multiple-choice questions carefully? Do you know how to choose wisely among alternative answers to questions? Test-taking skills and techniques are not a substitute for good study habits or an adequate grasp of the content and abilities measured in an examination. If you have a thorough understanding of the knowledge measured in an examination, however, good test-taking skills will enhance your overall performance.

To become oriented to test-taking skills that you can use in taking examinations such as *AssessTest* or licensure examinations, you need to know something about the language of multiple-choice questions. The question in its entirety is called a test item. The portion of the test item that poses the question or problem is called the stem. Potential answers to the question or problem posed are called options. In well-constructed multiple-choice items there is only one correct answer among the options supplied; the incorrect options are called distractors. Look at the following item and see if you can correctly label the item components.

The first step in the nursing process is:
1. Planning
2. Analyzing
3. Evaluation
4. Assessment

In this sample item, option **4** is correct; options **1, 2,** and **3** are the distractors. In this example the stem is in the form of an incomplete sentence, and each of the options could complete it. Stems may also be stated as questions. For instance, the stem could have read: "What is the first step in the nursing process?"

Remember that test questions are meant to measure your nursing knowledge. The items may be easy to read, but the answers to questions are not intended to be readily apparent. The questions draw on your ability to apply nursing knowledge from a variety of sources.

The following test-taking methods can increase your probability of choosing the correct answer to a question.

Read questions carefully. Scores on written tests are strongly affected by reading ability. In answering a test item, you should begin by carefully reading the stem and then asking yourself the following questions:

What is the question really asking?
Are there any key words?
What information relevant to answering this question is included in the stem?
How would I ask this question in my own words?
How would I answer this question in my own words?
After you have answered these questions, carefully read the options and then ask yourself the following questions:
Is there an option that is similar to the one I thought of?
Is this option the best, most complete answer to the question?

Deal with the question as it is stated, without reading anything into it or making assumptions about it. Answer the question asked, not the one you would like to answer. For simple recall items the self-questioning process will usually be completed quickly. For more complex items the self-questioning process may take longer, but it should assist you in clarifying the item and selecting the best response.

Eliminate clearly wrong or incorrect answers. Eliminate clearly incorrect, inappropriate, and unlikely answers to the question asked in the stem. By systematically eliminating distractors that are unlikely in the context of a given question, you increase the probability of selecting the correct answer. Eliminating obvious distractors also allows you more time to focus on the options that appear to be potentially sound answers to the question. Consider the following example:

The four levels of cognitive ability are:
1. Assessment, analysis, application, evaluation
2. Knowledge, comprehension, application, analysis
3. Knowledge, analysis, assessment, comprehension
4. Medical nursing, surgical nursing, obstetrical nursing, psychiatric nursing

Option **1** contains both cognitive levels and nursing behaviors, thus eliminating it from consideration. Option **4** is clearly inappropriate, as the choices are all clinical areas. Both options **2** and **3** contain levels of cognitive ability; however, option **3** includes assessment, which is a nursing behavior. Therefore option **2** is correct. By reducing the plausible options, you reduce the material to consider and increase the probability of selecting the correct option.

Identify similar options. When an item contains two or more options that are very similar in meaning, the successful test taker knows that all are correct, in which case it is a poor question, or that none is correct, which is more likely to be the case. The correct option will usually either include all the similar options or exclude them entirely.

In teaching new diabetics about their condition, it is important to focus on:
1. Dietary modifications
2. Use of exchange lists
3. Use of sugar substitutes
4. Their present understanding of diabetes

Options **1, 2,** and **3** deal only with the diabetic diet, involving no other aspect of diabetic teaching; it is impossible to select the most correct option because each represents an equally plausible, though limited, answer to the question. Option **4** is the best choice because it includes the other three options and is most complete. It therefore allows the other three options to be excluded as answers.

A child's intelligence is influenced by:
1. A variety of factors
2. Heredity and environment

3. Environment and experience
4. Education and economic factors

The most correct answer is option **1**. It includes the material covered by the other options, eliminating the need for an impossible choice, as each of the other options is only partially correct.

Identify answer (option) components. When an answer contains two or more parts, you can reduce the number of potentially correct answers by identifying one part as incorrect.

The nurse is aware that the signs of pregnancy-induced hypertension would include:
1. Proteinuria, hypotension, weight gain
2. Proteinuria, hypertension, weight gain
3. Ketonuria, hypotension, pitting edema
4. Ketonuria, hypertension, physiological edema

If you know, for instance, that pregnancy-induced hypertension does in fact cause hypertension, you can eliminate options **1** and **3** from consideration. If you know that pregnancy-induced hypertension causes protein in the urine rather than ketones you can eliminate option **4**. Therefore option **2** is correct.

Identify specific determiners. When the options of a test item contain words that are identical or similar to words in the stem, the alert test taker recognizes the similarities as clues about the likely answer to the question. The stem word that clues you to a similar word in the option or that limits potential options is known as a specific determiner.

The government agency responsible for administering the nursing practice act in each state is the:
1. Board of nursing
2. Board of regents
3. State nurses' association
4. State hospital association

Options **1** and **3** contain the closely related words *nurse* and *nursing*. The word *nursing*, used both in the stem and in item **1**, is a clue to the correct answer.

Identify words in the options that are closely associated with words in the stem. Be alert to words in the options that may be closely associated with but not identical to a word or words in the stem.

When a person develops symptoms of physical illness for which psychogenic factors act as causative agents, the resulting illness is classified as:
1. Dissociative
2. Compensatory
3. Psychophysiologic
4. Reaction formation

Option **3** ought to strike you as a likely answer, as it combines physical and psychologic factors, like those referred to in the stem.

Be alert to relevant information from earlier questions. Occasionally, information from one question may provide you with a clue for answering future questions.

A client has a nasogastric tube inserted after surgery. The nurse is aware that gastric suction can result in excessive loss of:
1. Protein enzymes
2. Energy carbohydrates
3. Water and electrolytes
4. Vitamins and minerals

If you know that the correct answer is option **3**, it may help you to answer a later question which asks:

Critical assessment of a client while an intestinal tube is draining should include observation for:
1. Edema
2. Nausea
3. Belching
4. Dehydration

The correct answer is option **4**. If you knew that excessive loss of water and electrolytes from nasogastric or intestinal suction may lead to dehydration, you could have used the clue provided in the early question to assist you in answering the later question.

Pay attention to specific details. The well-written multiple-choice question is precisely stated, providing you with only the information needed to make the question or problem clear and specific. Careful reading of details in the stem can provide you with important clues to the correct option.

A male client is told that he will no longer be able to ingest alcohol if he wants to live. To effect a change in the client's behavior while he is in the hospital, the nurse should attempt to:
1. Help the client set short-term dietary goals
2. Discuss his hopes and dreams for the future
3. Discuss the pathophysiology of the liver with him
4. Withhold approval until he agrees to stop drinking

The specific clause *to effect a change in the client's behavior while he is in the hospital* is critical. Option **2** is not really related to the client's alcoholism. Option **3** may be part of educating the alcoholic client, but you would not expect a behavioral change observable in the hospital to emerge from this discussion. Option **4** rejects the client as well as the client's behavior instead of only the client's behavior. Option **1**, the correct answer, could result in an observable behavioral change while the client is hospitalized; for example, the client could define ways to achieve short-term goals relating to diet and alcohol while in the hospital.

Identify key words. Certain key words in the stem, the options, or both should alert you to the need for caution in choosing your answer. Some of these key words are *all, never, only, must, no, none, always, except,* and *every.* These are strong words. They place special limitations and qualifications on potentially correct answers.

All of the following are services of the National Kidney Foundation except:
1. *Public education programs*
2. *Research about kidney disease*
3. *Fund-raising affairs for research activities*
4. *Identification of potential transplant recipients*

The stem contains two key words: *all* and *except.* They limit the choice of a correct answer to the one option that does not represent a service of the National Kidney Foundation. When *except, not,* or a phrase such as *all but one of the following* appears in the stem, the inappropriate option is the correct answer; in this instance, option **4.** Also be on guard when you see one of the key words in an option; it may limit the contexts in which such an option would be correct.

If the options in an item do not seem to make sense because more than one is correct, reread the question; you may have missed some key words in the stem.

The nurse teaches a client with diabetes mellitus how to perform foot care. The nurse would recognize that further teaching was necessary when the client states:
1. *"I will visit my podiatrist every 6 weeks."*
2. *"I will check my feet daily for signs of pressure."*
3. *"I will wash and gently dry my feet at least twice a day."*
4. *"I will wear only nylon or nylon and cotton–mixed socks."*

In this question the stem is really asking which response by the client is incorrect and needs to be changed by further education. Options **1, 2,** and **3** demonstrate an appropriate level of understanding, whereas option **4** is incorrect and demonstrates a need for further teaching.

Watch for grammatical inconsistencies. If one or more of the options is not grammatically consistent with the stem, the alert test taker can frequently eliminate these distractors. When the stem is in the form of an incomplete sentence, each option should complete the sentence in a grammatically correct way. The correct option must be consistent with the form of the question. If the question demands a response in the singular, plural options usually can be safely eliminated.

The nurse is aware that initiating communication with a client who is deaf will be facilitated by:
1. *The use of gestures*
2. *Facing the client while speaking*
3. *Find out if the client has a hearing aid*
4. *Speaking loudly often helps clients hear*

Options **3** and **4** do not complete the sentence in a grammatically consistent way and can be safely eliminated, leaving the choice between options **1** and **2.** Option **1** may help once the client and nurse have established a nonverbal mode of communication, but gestures can frequently be misunderstood initially, leaving option **2** as the best choice.

Make educated guesses. On the computerized NCLEX, you will not be able to go on to the next question until an answer is selected for the present question. You can generally eliminate one or more of the distractors by using partial knowledge and the methods just listed. The elimination process increases your chances of selecting the correct option from those remaining. Elimination of 2 distractors on a 4-option multiple-choice item increases your probability of selecting the correct answer from 25% to 50%. First use educated guesses, then move to pure guessing. You have at least a 1 in 4 (25%) chance of guessing the correct answer.

Use the rules of test wisdom

- Study! There is no escape! All the test-taking skills and techniques will be of little use if you do not have a good grasp of the content to be tested.
- Follow all written or oral directions for taking the test.
- Read carefully and think about what you read.
- Remember that every word in a question matters. Attend to detail.
- Answer the question asked.
- Put questions and answers in your own words to test your comprehension.
- Read each option carefully and compare options, looking for similarities and conflicts among them.
- Eliminate obviously incorrect options quickly so you can spend time on more plausible ones.
- Relate options to the question asked.
- Look for clues in the question that might lead you to the correct option.
- Watch for key words such as *all, never,* and *only* in both the questions and the options.
- Assess grammatical and logical consistency between the question and each option. Eliminate options that are inconsistent.
- Attempt to recall clues from previous questions.
- Be aware of cultural differences and moral biases, but do not base your answers on your personal beliefs and practices.
- Avoid selecting answers that reflect specific hospital policies, rules, or regulations.
- Be alert for questions that require you to determine priorities among four plausible options. State criteria for determining priorities to yourself.
- Make educated guesses.
- Select the option that provides the most complete, appropriate answer to the question.

- Stay with your first answer unless you have a very specific reason to change it.

Use this opportunity to learn how to manage your test-taking time

Because many examinations have specified time limits (even the NCLEX/CAT has a maxium time of 5 hours), you will need to pace yourself during the testing period and work as quickly and accurately as possible. On examinations where the exact number of questions and the allotted time is known, it is helpful to estimate the time that can be spent on each item and still complete the examination in the allotted time. Obtain this figure by dividing the testing time by the number of items on the test. For example, with a 75 minute testing period and 75 items, an average of 1 minute per item will be the appropriate pace.

Although certain questions will be more difficult than others and will require more time, spending too much time on these difficult items may compromise your overall score. On the *AssessTest* you can make a mark next to the item you cannot answer and go on. After you have answered all the questions you can answer easily, return to the marked items. Be sure to erase any extraneous marks near your answers. If time remains, it is useful to review all your answers, making sure you have marked them correctly.

NOTE: For the NCLEX-RN CAT, you will be unable to return to any previous question, and every question must be answered before moving on.

Do not be pressured into finishing early. Do not rush! Typically, students who achieve higher scores use all the time available.

Use this opportunity to build your test-taking confidence

You should feel confident and competent if you have studied and reviewed the content to be tested and you are armed with methods for reading and answering questions. Questions that seem complicated at first glance can often be answered with the "educated guess." Remain calm and confident. Your emotional state is vitally important when thinking about, preparing for, and taking any test. Think positively.

Use the *AssessTest* as a learning experience

The *AssessTest* is a valuable evaluating tool designed to test your level of knowledge. However, it is equally as valuable in providing information from incorrect answers. By studying the rationales for the incorrect selections, you will have an excellent opportunity to learn from your mistakes. In addition, the computer analysis of your performance that you receive will identify areas of strength and weakness, information that will assist you when focusing study time.

COMPUTER EVALUATION

After your completed answer sheet has been processed and scored, you will receive a computerized evaluation of your test results. The evaluation will provide specific data regarding your overall performance and your performance in each of the categories measured by *AssessTest*. You will also receive a booklet of "Answers and Rationales" that has been designed to help the testee understand why the correct answer was correct and the reason each of the incorrect answers was incorrect for each question on the *AssessTest*. The booklet also indicates the classifications for each question.

The introduction to this booklet explains how to interpret your computer analysis and how best to use the data on the report to design a personal study plan. Using this information along with the questions in the *AssessTest* and the "Answers and Rationales" booklet will help you learn from your mistakes and make the most of your *AssessTest* experience.

AssessTest

DIRECTIONS FOR TAKING *AssessTest*

To gain the maximum benefit from this experience, it is vital that you follow *precisely* and *completely* the directions for taking the examination and returning the answer sheet. The personal computer analysis you receive will give you a true picture of your abilities if you have taken the test under conditions that are as controlled as possible and if your answers reflect your best efforts. Be sure that you have not overlooked or misunderstood any test directions and that the rules and procedures of the examination are absolutely clear to you before beginning.

Materials needed

You will need the following materials:
1. Your test manual
2. Answer sheet (included with manual)
3. A number 2 (soft lead) pencil (Do not use a ballpoint pen, colored lead, or any other type of writing instrument. The tests are machine scored, and only answers marked with a soft-lead pencil will be recorded.)
4. An eraser

Time needed

There are four comprehensive tests. Each test consists of 75 questions. It is assumed that you will use about 1 minute per question. Allow 75 minutes for each comprehensive test.

How to take the test

1. Read each question *carefully*.
2. Go through the test you are working on once, answering the questions you feel sure about first.
3. Go back over the test a second time and answer the remaining questions. Answer *all* the questions. If you must guess, eliminate the obviously incorrect answers first and base your guess on the remaining alternatives. You will receive feedback based on the responses you select.
4. Because the computer printout will keep track of *only* the questions you answered incorrectly, you should circle your answers directly on the test booklet as well as marking your answer sheet. By circling the answers in the test booklet, you will have a record of all of your responses. *The analysis you receive will not include a record of your correct responses.*

NOTE: Your score on *AssessTest* is based on the number of questions you answer correctly. The number of questions missed is subtracted from the total number of questions (300) to determine your score. Because *AssessTest* is designed to help you identify your strengths and weaknesses, it is to your advantage to answer all the questions. Be sure you understand the grading system when taking examinations. Guide your test-taking approach accordingly.

How To Complete The Answer Sheet

Read these directions carefully *before* filling out the answer sheet. Use only a number 2 (soft lead) pencil. Make heavy, black marks. Erase thoroughly if you change an answer. Record answers in designated spaces only. Do not make any other marks on the answer sheet.

Side 1 (personal data)

Please answer all questions and print clearly.
1. *Your name.* Print your name in the row of empty boxes provided, skipping one space between words. As you enter each letter, darken the oval with the corresponding printed letter in the column directly below it. Do not make dots, crosses, circles, Xs, or lines; fill in only a single oval for each letter.
2. *Your mailing address.* Fill in the boxes as you did with your name, marking appropriate letters or numbers beneath those you have entered. Use the following abbreviations in the street number and name and city or town as necessary:

APARTMENT	APT
AVENUE	AVE
BOULEVARD	BLVD
BOX	BX
CENTER	CTR
CIRCLE	CIR
CITY	CTY
COLLEGE	COL
COMMUNITY	CMTY

COUNTY	CNTY	CALIFORNIA	CA
COURT	CT	COLORADO	CO
DRIVE	DR	CONNECTICUT	CT
EAST	E	DELAWARE	DE
FLOOR	FLR	DISTRICT OF COLUMBIA	DC
FORT	FT	FLORIDA	FL
GARDEN	GDN	GEORGIA	GA
GENERAL	GEN	HAWAII	HI
HEALTH	HLTH	IDAHO	ID
HEIGHTS	HTS	ILLINOIS	IL
HIGHWAY	HWY	INDIANA	IN
HOSPITAL	HSP	IOWA	IA
INSTITUTE	INST	KANSAS	KS
JUNCTION	JCT	KENTUCKY	KY
LAKE	LK	LOUISIANA	LA
LANE	LN	MAINE	ME
MEDICAL	MED	MARYLAND	MD
MEMORIAL	MEM	MASSACHUSETTS	MA
MOUNT	MT	MICHIGAN	MI
MOUNTAIN	MT	MINNESOTA	MN
NORTH	N	MISSISSIPPI	MS
PARK	PK	MISSOURI	MO
PARKWAY	PKWY	MONTANA	MT
PIKE	PI	NEBRASKA	NE
PLACE	PL	NEVADA	NV
POINT	PT	NEW HAMPSHIRE	NH
PORT	PT	NEW JERSEY	NJ
POST OFFICE	PO	NEW MEXICO	NM
REGIONAL	REG	NEW YORK	NY
ROAD	RD	NORTH CAROLINA	NC
ROUTE	RT	NORTH DAKOTA	ND
SCHOOL	SCH	OHIO	OH
SERVICE	SVC	OKLAHOMA	OK
SOUTH	S	OREGON	OR
STATION	STA	PENNSYLVANIA	PA
STREET	ST	RHODE ISLAND	RI
TECHNICAL	TECH	SOUTH CAROLINA	SC
TERRACE	TR	SOUTH DAKOTA	SD
TRAIL	TR	TENNESSEE	TN
TRAILER	TRLR	TEXAS	TX
TURNPIKE	TPKE	UTAH	UT
UNIVERSITY	UNIV	VERMONT	VT
WARD	WD	VIRGINIA	VA
WAY	WY	WASHINGTON	WA
WEST	W	WEST VIRGINIA	WV
		WISCONSIN	WI
		WYOMING	WY
		PUERTO RICO	PR
		VIRGIN ISLANDS	VI

In the two boxes labeled *State* or *Province* enter one of the following abbreviations and fill in the ovals corresponding to the letters you have entered:

ALABAMA	AL	ALBERTA	AB
ALASKA	AK	BRITISH COLUMBIA	BC
ARIZONA	AZ	MANITOBA	MB
ARKANSAS	AR	NEW BRUNSWICK	NB

NORTHWEST TERRITORIES	NT
NOVA SCOTIA	NS
ONTARIO	ON
PRINCE EDWARD ISLAND	PE
PROVINCE OF QUEBEC	PQ
SASKATCHEWAN	SK
YUKON TERRITORY	YT
LABRADOR	LB
NEWFOUNDLAND	NF
NOT LISTED	NL

Mark the appropriate space in the box labeled *Country of Current Mailing Address.*

3. *Demographic questions.* Answer all questions on the lower part of the form. Select only one response for each question (the one that is most nearly correct). This information will be used only for statistical purposes and will in no way affect your test results.
4. *School name.* If you are still in school or have recently graduated and have not yet taken the licensure examination, indicate your nursing school. If you are a licensed nurse in practice, indicate the name of the hospital or institution with which you are affiliated. If you are taking the test as a required part of a review course not conducted by your nursing school, indicate the name of the course.
5. *Date.* Fill in the date on which you complete the test.

If your state or province is not listed and you enter NL in the boxes, complete your mailing address on Side 2 of your answer sheet.

Side 2 (answer sheet)

You are now ready to begin the first test. Fill out the answer sheet as follows:

1. Print your address at the top of the answer sheet in the spaces provided.
2. Turn to Comprehensive Examination 1 in the booklet.
3. Start with the space marked 1 under Test 1 on your answer sheet (Side 2). Mark only one answer per question. Use a number 2 (soft lead) pencil. Make heavy, dark marks. Erase changes completely. Be sure you put your answers in the correct spaces on your answer sheet. Check question numbers as you go.
4. Complete all four tests. Try to finish at least one whole test at a sitting.

Returning the answer sheet

When you have completed all four tests, enter the date of completion on Side 1. Return the completed answer sheet to your instructor, who will mail all documents for scoring. **Do not mail your own answer sheet unless you are taking this text as an individual.**

DIRECTIONS FOR GROUP ADMINISTRATION OF *AssessTest*

To obtain a statistical summary of group performance, your group must include 10 or more participants. You may divide the test administration into whatever time periods are convenient for you, but it is suggested that at least one test be completed per sitting. Each test requires 75 minutes for completion. The answer sheet is to be filled in as described on pp. 16 to 18.

To obtain the computer profile of your group's performance, you *must* send all of the students' answer sheets in for scoring at one time. Answer sheets should be mailed first class in *one* envelope. A pre-addressed envelope is provided with your order. Answer sheets should be stacked, unclipped, unstapled, and unfolded.

Mail to:
Mosby's RN *AssessTest*
Professional Testing Corporation
1211 Avenue of the Americas
15th Floor
New York, NY 10036

Please be sure the envelope bears adequate postage.

A cover sheet must be completed and placed on top of the answer sheets. A cover sheet is provided with your order. If it has been misplaced, use the copy on p. 19. Please fill out the cover sheet completely and neatly. Be sure to indicate the type of program: diploma, associate degree, or baccalaureate. *All the tests for your group must be returned together.* This is the only way that you can obtain your institutional profile with the summary document of your group's performance. The individual test results may be returned *either* to your institution or to the individual student. **If you do not indicate where individual results should be sent, they will be mailed to the institution.** The institutional summary will be mailed to the institution. Any questions should be directed to Kathy Rosler, Customer Quality Support, Mosby–Year Book, Inc., St. Louis, Missouri. Write or call toll-free (800) 633-6699.

COVER SHEET
1997
UNSECURED *AssessTest*

GROUP-ADMINISTERED RN *AssessTest*

Please enclose this sheet with the answer documents for your group. Do not fold the answer documents or insert them in the individual return envelopes. All forms should be batched together in one envelope for group processing and mailed to:

MOSBY'S RN AssessTest – GROUP TESTING
Professional Testing Corporation
15th Floor
1211 Avenue of the Americas
New York, NY 10036

The total number of answer sheets included for this group is _____

Please indicate your preference: ❏ The individual student   ❏ The institution
(Check only *one*)

NOTE: If a box is not checked, test results will be sent to the institution.

Mail institutional profile (and individual results if "the institution" is checked above) to:

Name _____

Title _____

Institution _____

Type of institution: ❏ Associate degree   ❏ Baccalaureate   ❏ Diploma

Address _____

_____

City _____

State _____ Zip code _____

Phone _____
(area code)

Today's date _____

PLEASE DO NOT WRITE IN THIS BOX - FOR OFFICE USE ONLY	
Date Received:	Date Scanned:
Number Received:	Date Mailed:

Instructions for group administration of AssessTest

- You may divide test administration into whatever time periods are convenient for you, but it is suggested that at least one test be completed per sitting.
- Each test requires about 1¼ hours for completion.
- Ten or more participants constitute a "group." The Institutional Profile (the summary of a group's performance) will not be prepared for groups of less than ten participants.
- Answer documents are to be filled out as described in detail on pp. 16-18 in the AssessTest booklet. Participants are instructed to:
  ____ Use a number 2 (soft lead) pencil in filling out answer document
  ____ Erase thoroughly any stray marks or changed answers on the answer documents
  ____ Print clearly when required
  ____ Fill out all blanks on Side 1 of the answer document, including name, address, demographic questions, and booklet number (found on the cover of the AssessTest booklet)

Mailing instructions for group administration of AssessTest

- *All* answer documents must be submitted for scoring at one time. All answer documents should be mailed first class in a single envelope. Please use the envelope provided.
- Answer documents should be stacked, unclipped, unstapled, and unfolded.
- The cover sheet (back of this sheet) should be placed on top of the answer sheets.
- Be sure to fill out the cover sheet accurately, indicating:
  ____ Where individual results are to be mailed (to the individual or to the institution)
  ____ The name, address, and phone number of the instructor and institution
  ____ The type of nursing program (associate degree, diploma, baccalaureate)
- Sufficient postage should be affixed to the envelope

Return Policy

- ALL UNUSED TESTS MUST BE RETURNED WITHIN 90 DAYS OF RECEIPT. CREDIT WILL NOT BE ISSUED FOR THOSE TESTS WHICH HAVE HAD THE POLYWRAP REMOVED.

ISBN 0-8151-8507-3

Comprehensive examination 1

1. The nurse is aware that the procedure that is used to help evaluate the pregnancy of an Rh-sensitized woman is:
   1. Ultrasonography
   2. Amniotic fluid analysis
   3. RhoGAM response testing
   4. Maternal bilirubin evaluation

2. The nurse adds the nursing diagnosis "Activity intolerance" to the nursing care plan of a 3-month-old admitted with cystic fibrosis. To help alleviate this nursing diagnosis for a 3-month-old the nurse should:
   1. Restrict visitors to reduce environmental stimuli
   2. Promote weight gain by providing pureed foods
   3. Conserve energy by providing a quiet environment for sleep
   4. Provide for rest times by performing only one nursing intervention per hour

3. The nurse prepares a 4-year-old for a bone marrow aspiration by:
   1. Starting to explain 2 days before what will happen and why
   2. Allowing the child to choose the site preferred for the procedure
   3. Warning the child well in advance that it will be painful and it is good to cry
   4. Waiting until just before the procedure and giving a quick but complete explanation

4. A voiding cystourethrogram is ordered for a 3-year-old boy after a urinary tract infection. The mother tells the nurse that she feels this is unnecessary, because her older daughter had a urinary infection last year and the procedure was not done. The nurse should explain that:
   1. The mother may be right and the nurse will question the physician about this order
   2. Urinary infections in boys are more likely to be related to anomalies of the urinary tract
   3. This is a new test and was probably not available when her daughter had the urinary infection
   4. Urinary tract infections in girls are related to the female anatomy rather than to the presence of anomalies

5. The nurse is taking a history from a client with the dual diagnoses of major depression and polysubstance abuse. Considering this client's dual diagnoses, the nurse would not be surprised if this client stated:
   1. "I kept hearing these strange voices."
   2. "While I was in detox, I tried to commit suicide."
   3. "Now that I am in the hospital, I feel energized."
   4. "You seem like a trustworthy person, so I'll tell you everything."

6. When relating with a client experiencing severe anxiety, it would be most helpful for the nurse to:
   1. Speak in short sentences and give concise instructions
   2. Explore with the client the underlying dynamics of anxiety
   3. Carefully explain in detail the treatment plans that have been developed
   4. Urge the client to concentrate on developing better interpersonal relationships

7. Following surgical repair of a hip fracture with an internal fixation device, the nurse plans to help restore normal anatomic function by positioning the affected extremity in:
   1. Slight hip flexion
   2. External rotation
   3. Moderate abduction
   4. Normal body alignment

8. A baby is born in the 28th week of pregnancy and weighs 850 g. There is variable immaturity in all body systems. It is essential for the nurse to assist the mother in understanding the possible problems a preterm newborn may experience. These problems could include:
   1. Macrosomia
   2. Phenylketonuria
   3. Muscular dystrophy
   4. Intraventricular hemorrhage

9. A client, 39-weeks gestation, is admitted in labor. This client is an insulin-dependent diabetic of 10-years duration. When planning care for this client following childbirth, the nurse knows that insulin requirements will decrease because of:
   1. Placental insulinase
   2. The client's NPO status
   3. Prolonged absorption of glucose
   4. Reduction in HPL (human placental lactogen)

10. The nurse is aware that transference is the:
    1. Nurse's partly unconscious or conscious emotional reaction to the client
    2. Process used to find equilibrium between oneself and one's environment
    3. Client's unconscious assignment to the nurse of feelings originally meant for others
    4. Process of auto-diagnosis or self-awareness that develops and expands with psychotherapy

11. When planning care to meet the nutritional needs of a lactating mother, the nurse should instruct the client to increase her intake of:
    1. Fat
    2. Iron
    3. Calories
    4. Vitamin A

12. A 1-month-old is admitted after 32 hours of vomiting and diarrhea. The nurse assesses the infant for physical signs of dehydration by checking for:
    1. Periorbital edema
    2. A bulging fontanel
    3. The presence of tears when the infant is crying
    4. The degree of moisture of the buccal mucous membranes

13. The nurse is giving care to an 18-month-old in Bryant traction. Part of the nursing intervention will involve being sure that the:
    1. Infant's body is lying completely flat on the mattress
    2. Ace bandage is rarely disturbed without a physician's order
    3. Antibiotic ointment is applied to the skeletal pins twice a day
    4. Infant's buttocks are raised off the mattress enough to fit a hand under them

14. The discharge teaching plan for a child recovering from nephrosis should include teaching the parents that the child should not be given routine immunizations while still taking:
    1. Aspirin
    2. Ampicillin
    3. Prednisone
    4. Ferrous sulfate

15. The nurse is aware that the children who are most likely to have an IQ within the normal range are children born with:
    1. Cri du chat
    2. Trisomy 18
    3. Down syndrome
    4. Turner syndrome

16. The nurse is caring for a 4-year-old who sustained burns over 30% of the trunk and arms. During the initial and acute emergent phase the nurse would immediately report:
    1. A pulse rate of 110
    2. A decrease in bowel sounds
    3. A rectal temperature of 101° F
    4. A urine output less than 1 to 2 ml/kg per hour

17. Following a coronary artery bypass graft (CABG), a client has an elevated mean arterial pressure (MAP) of 130 mmHg. Drug therapy postoperatively would probably include:
    1. Norepinephrine (Levophed)
    2. Sodium nitroprusside (Nipride)
    3. Isoproterenol hydrochloride (Isuprel)
    4. Dobutamine hydrochloride (Dobutrex)

18. A client with unstable angina is receiving a continuous infusion of nitroglycerin. The nurse should monitor the client's:
    1. Heart rate
    2. Blood pressure
    3. Potassium level
    4. CK isoenzymes

19. The nurse should expect that the stools of a client with ulcerative colitis would be:
    1. Foul smelling
    2. Green mucusy
    3. Bloody diarrhea
    4. A puttylike color

20. A client is admitted to the emergency department with an acute myocardial infarction. Priority care by the nurse in the emergency room should include:
    1. Administering atropine
    2. Providing for pain control
    3. Reducing the family's anxiety
    4. Preparing the client for invasive monitoring

21. A client with acute myocardial infarction is receiving alteplase t-PA/heparin therapy. The nurse should assess for:
    1. Hypertension
    2. GU or GI bleeding
    3. Macular degeneration
    4. A decreased partial thromboplastin time

22. When assigning points on the Apgar score, a heart rate of 130 beats per minute should receive a score of:
    1. 0
    2. 1
    3. 2
    4. 3

23. A client diagnosed with AIDS has developed sepsis. Trimethoprim-sulfamethoxazole (Bactrim) is ordered intravenously in divided doses. The nurse should withhold the drug and notify the physician if the client:
    1. Is confused and depressed
    2. Has a skin rash on the face
    3. Expresses a dislike of intravenous medication
    4. Has old scars over the veins on the arms and legs

24. A client is admitted to the surgical ICU following triple-vessel coronary artery bypass graft surgery. Atrial fibrillation with a ventricular rate of 150/min is documented on the monitor. The nurse should initially:
    1. Attempt defibrillation
    2. Assess blood pressure
    3. Prepare prescribed atropine
    4. Administer a bolus of ordered lidocaine

25. Because of the intestinal structure and function associated with ulcerative colitis, a 22-year-old will need psychologic support to satisfactorily meet Erikson's developmental crisis of young adulthood, which is:
    1. Intimacy versus isolation
    2. Ego integrity versus despair
    3. Identity versus role diffusion
    4. Generativity versus stagnation

26. A client who has had a heart transplant is to receive oral cyclosporin (Sandimmune). When instructing the client about this drug, the nurse should tell the client that the drug:
    1. Should not be diluted before administering
    2. May be stored in any dark container, although styrofoam is preferred
    3. Can cause hypotension, and blood pressure should be monitored at frequent intervals
    4. Will interfere with kidney function, and blood studies need to be performed at established intervals

27. A client who is to undergo a carotid endarterectomy asks the nurse to describe this procedure. The nurse would be correct in stating that a carotid endarterectomy involves:
    1. Removal of the dura mater layer of the carotid artery
    2. Excision of a segment of the intimal layer of the carotid artery
    3. Inflation of a balloon in the artery to break up atherosclerotic plaques
    4. Anastomosis of a segment of a saphenous vein to the stenosed carotid artery

28. When ambulating a client following a press-fit hip replacement, the nurse should:
    1. Caution the client about weight bearing on the affected side
    2. Allow the client to assume weight bearing on both legs for balance
    3. Delay active ambulation until hip x-rays show evidence of bone growth
    4. Remove the thigh-high elastic stockings because ambulation will prevent phlebitis

29. A client has difficulty sleeping throughout the night, waking often and getting up to check the windows and doors to see that they are locked. This is an example of:
    1. A simple phobia
    2. A compulsive act
    3. An obsessive thought
    4. The use of displacement

30. When developing a plan of care for a child with sickle cell crisis (pain episode), the nurse considers the fact that the slowed circulation present during sickle cell crisis can cause:
    1. Hemolysis
    2. Kidney failure
    3. Cardiac failure
    4. Hemolytic anemia

31. A 48-year-old ataxic and irritable female is admitted with traumatic injuries. When asked how this occurred, the client's husband states, "She tripped over the cat while coming down the staircase about six hours ago." During the assessment the nurse observes hand tremors, peripheral neuritis, a BP of 160/100, and a pulse rate of 95. The nurse determines the need to obtain further information regarding:
    1. Alcohol abuse
    2. Nerve damage

3. Nicotine abuse
4. Cardiac disease

32. A newborn infant is examined in the nursery. The nurse recognizes that congenital hip dysplasia is likely to be present when it is noted that there is:
    1. Inability to fully extend the legs
    2. Limited abduction of both legs when flexed and abducted
    3. A tendency for the infant to hold the legs in a flexed position
    4. Free movement of both thighs when the legs are flexed and abducted

33. After initial home treatment is unsuccessful, a client is hospitalized for treatment of pregnancy-induced hypertension. The client is placed on bed rest with bathroom privileges. Because of her elevated blood pressure, an appropriate nursing diagnosis for this client would be:
    1. Risk for loneliness
    2. Activity intolerance
    3. Impaired gas exchange
    4. Altered tissue perfusion

34. Terbutaline sulfate (Brethine), a drug used to halt preterm labor, is classified as:
    1. A sedative
    2. An anticonvulsive
    3. A beta-adrenergic
    4. An antihypertensive

35. The nurse will be able to positively evaluate a parent's knowledge of oral iron supplement administration when the parent states:
    1. "I'll give my child the iron pill once a week."
    2. "I'll give the iron pill with a cup of tea with milk."
    3. "I'll brush my child's teeth after I give the liquid iron."
    4. "I don't have to worry about poisoning, because iron is nontoxic."

36. An 18-month-old child received partial thickness burns to the trunk after being scalded by hot coffee. The nurse's initial assessment would probably reveal:
    1. Burns with blackened edges
    2. Calmness of a shocklike quality
    3. Red, dry skin on the child's chest
    4. A child screaming and writhing in pain

37. A newborn is scheduled to have surgery to correct a pyloric stenosis. The nurse establishes that the goal highest in priority would be:
    1. Correcting dehydration
    2. Maintaining body weight
    3. Providing preoperative teaching
    4. Establishing a central venous line

38. A 5-year-old was admitted to the hospital with a diagnosis of acute lymphocytic leukemia, which was confirmed after a bone marrow aspiration. The child is scheduled to have a lumbar puncture done to:
    1. Monitor the intracranial pressure
    2. Prevent the child from developing meningitis
    3. Detect any infiltration of the central nervous system
    4. Determine the present stage of the disease process

39. A 5-year-old with chicken pox experiences a febrile seizure and is brought to the emergency room. The nurse determines the nursing diagnosis of highest priority to be:
    1. Pain related to itching
    2. Risk for injury related to a neurologic event
    3. Knowledge deficit (of parents) related to fever
    4. Risk for infection related to infectious varicella

40. A client with congestive heart failure is receiving Lasix and low-dose intravenous nitroglycerin. The nurse can evaluate the effectiveness of treatment by:
    1. An increase in blood pressure
    2. An increase in serum potassium
    3. A decrease in ventricular dysrhythmias
    4. A decrease in the pulmonary capillary wedge pressure

41. The nursing intervention with the highest priority in the early management of a client with a narcotic overdose would be:
    1. Requesting a psychologic evaluation
    2. Continuing to observe the size of pupils
    3. Documenting the extent of tendon reflexes
    4. Auscultating the chest to assess for pulmonary edema

42. A client is admitted to the coronary care unit following a percutaneous transluminal coronary angioplasty (PTCA). The nurse should assess for acute vessel closure by:
    1. Monitoring PTT results
    2. Checking for a rise in CK isoenzymes
    3. Monitoring the ST segment continuously
    4. Observing for a decrease in urinary output

43. The nurse identifies that the client with renal failure is accepting the need for dialysis treatments when the client states:
    1. "I am only dependent on dialysis until function is restored."
    2. "Yes, I've been ill, but with the aid of dialysis I will meet life head on."
    3. "Herman, that's what I call my machine, is part of my life and is my best friend."
    4. "My family will need to make few changes in their lifestyle or way of living on my behalf."

44. Postoperatively, a client who is allergic to narcotics has electrodes for a transcutaneous elective nerve stimulation (TENS) attached on both sides of the incision before the wound is covered. To safely help control pain the nurse should:
    1. Change electrodes every shift
    2. Advise the client to avoid using an electric razor
    3. Unplug the unit from the electrical outlet q 2 hours
    4. Adjust the frequency and amplitude controls on the TENS unit

45. After surgery for uterine cancer, it is determined that adjuvant radiation therapy is needed because of abdominal metastases. The client asks why the treatments are scheduled for a date almost 5 weeks in the future. The nurse's most appropriate response would be:
    1. "If treatment is begun earlier, it could interfere with the healing process following your surgery."
    2. "The delay will schedule therapy at the time the cancer cells are most active and thus most easily destroyed."
    3. "You may not be able to take all the treatments now, and once treatments are started they must not be interrupted."
    4. "It will give you time to improve your general state of health so you will derive the greatest benefit from the treatment."

46. A client admitted in an alcoholic stupor develops increased tremors, irritability, hypertension, and fever. The nurse should be alert for impending:
    1. Delirium tremens
    2. Esophageal varices
    3. Korsakoff's psychosis
    4. Wernicke's encephalopathy

47. A family member's repeated attempts at excusing and covering up a client's drinking problem are indicative of the behavior associated with:
    1. Guilt
    2. Denial
    3. Co-dependency
    4. A drinking problem

48. The nursing plan for counseling an adult client who has HIV/AIDS should begin with:
    1. Exploring priorities as seen by the client
    2. Discussing nutritional factors related to HIV
    3. Including the family in health care decisions
    4. Teaching the client the necessity for safe sex

49. A client on the mental health unit states, "I am the president of the world's largest computer firm." The nurse recognizes the client:
    1. Has delusions of persecution
    2. May be the president of a large computer firm
    3. Has a low self esteem and deliberately distorts reality
    4. Is trying to adapt to a low self concept by being someone important

50. A client is placed on cancer chemotherapy every 6 weeks following surgery to remove a cancerous tumor of the breast. Two of the drugs, methotrexate and 5-flurouracil, are antimetabolites whose cytoxic activity primarily occurs at the S phase of the cell cycle. The medication the nurse should expect to administer to the client on this chemotherapy regimen is:
    1. Leucovorin (folic acid)
    2. Theragram (multivitamins)
    3. Premarin (estrogen replacement)
    4. Testosterone (androgen replacement)

51. A newborn has a myelomeningocele and is scheduled for surgery. The nursing action that best facilitates parent-child relationships in the preoperative period would be to:

1. Allow the parents to cuddle the child in their arms
2. Teach the parents how to bathe the child after surgery
3. Encourage the parents to stroke and comfort the child
4. Demonstrate the prone position feeding technique to the parents

52. While the nurse is administering care to a client in acute renal failure, the client says, "My doctor says that I am going to get insulin. Do I also have diabetes?" The response by the nurse that would best demonstrate an understanding of the use of insulin in acute renal failure is:
    1. "Why don't you ask your doctor that question on the next visit?"
    2. "No, the insulin will help your body handle a chemical called potassium."
    3. "You probably had an elevated blood sugar level, so your doctor is being cautious."
    4. "No, but insulin will reduce the toxins in your blood by lowering your metabolic rate."

53. A 50-year-old unmarried client who found a lump in her breast consults a surgeon, who recommends a mammogram and biopsy of her breast. The client asks the nurse why a mammogram and a biopsy are necessary. The nurse should reply:
    1. "The mammogram will help the surgeon to further evaluate the breast mass."
    2. "It is the routine of surgeons in the hospital to do a mammogram before a biopsy."
    3. "The surgeon probably wants to know if a cancerous mass should be expected during the biopsy."
    4. "A mammogram is always needed prior to a biopsy in order to detect the exact size of the mass."

54. A male client in the mental health clinic tells the nurse that he can no longer function at his job because his mind is constantly thinking that something bad will happen to his wife and baby, even though he knows that this is foolish. The nurse identifies this response as:
    1. A phobia
    2. An obsession
    3. Hypochondriasis
    4. Compulsive behavior

55. A client is placed on a continuous passive motion machine following a total knee replacement. Postoperative nursing care will include:
    1. Placement of a trochanter roll
    2. The use of an abduction pillow
    3. Special wedges to prevent dislocation
    4. Observation for bleeding at the operative site

56. When developing a nursing diagnosis for a pregnant, low-income female with 5 children who has an iron-deficiency anemia, the nurse should consider:
    1. Fatigue related to demands of a large family
    2. Altered role performance related to demands of a large family
    3. Activity intolerance related to physiologic changes of pregnancy
    4. Altered nutrition: less than body requirements related to inadequate dietary intake

57. The laboratory value for a hospitalized 8-year-old that would indicate the need for immediate intervention is:
    1. Sodium 138 mg
    2. Chloride 104 mEq
    3. Potassium 5.8 mEq
    4. Hemoglobin 11.6 g/dl

58. A client who suspects that she is pregnant is to have a pregnancy test done on her urine. The nurse:
    1. Teaches her to collect a mid-stream specimen
    2. Advises her to test any random specimen of urine
    3. Tells her that she will be collecting a 24-hour specimen
    4. Instructs her to fast after bedtime, prior to collection of the specimen

59. A client is to have arthroscopy under local anesthesia. The nurse instructs the client to void just before surgery. The primary reason for this request is to:
    1. Minimize vagal nerve stimulation
    2. Prevent surgical damage to a full bladder
    3. Prevent contamination of the operative site
    4. Increase the client's comfort during the procedure

60. A client returns from reconstructive surgery of the knee with a portable wound drain. After emptying the portable collecting reservoir, the nurse should:
    1. Pump the reservoir repeatedly to increase the suction
    2. Caution the client that it will be painful when the suction is reapplied
    3. Compress the reservoir and record the amount and character of the drainage
    4. Leave the drain clamped for 30 minutes before returning it to the suction mode

61. The factor which would most likely predispose a client to the development of shock following a fracture of the femur is:
    1. Pooling of the blood in the lower legs
    2. Generalized vasoconstriction in the lower extremities
    3. Loss of blood into soft tissues surrounding the fracture
    4. Depression of the adrenal gland by toxins released at the injury

62. The tests that the nurse would expect to be ordered after a client has returned from a permanent pacemaker implantation would be:
    1. A chest x-ray and an EKG
    2. Cardiac enzymes and an EKG
    3. A chest x-ray and blood cultures
    4. Cardiac enzymes and a chest x-ray

63. A client with a history of diabetes mellitus delivers a baby girl. The assessment of an infant of a diabetic mother would likely reveal that the baby's:
    1. Appearance is puffy and Cushingoid-like
    2. Size is consistent with the gestational age
    3. Head appears large as compared to the trunk
    4. Skin is parchmentlike and vernix is in the skin folds only

64. The best initial intervention for the nurse to use to establish trust with a newly admitted hostile, suspicious, delusional client would be,"I am your nurse:
    1. Come with me to your room."
    2. I'd like to show you to your room."
    3. Come and tell me when you want to go to your room."
    4. Let me review your chart, then I'll show you to your room."

65. A female is being seen in the crisis center after the sudden death of her husband and the loss of her job. The client has no immediate family except for a 15-year-old son. Her greatest fear is how she will pay the rent and other expenses and support him on her unemployment insurance. The nurse, in planning with the client, should first suggest that:
    1. The client go out and get another job
    2. The son get a part-time job after school
    3. The client share her concerns with her son
    4. The nurse and the client make out a monthly budget together

66. The arterial blood gases of a client with COPD deteriorate, and respiratory failure is impending. The nurse should assess the client for:
    1. Cyanosis
    2. Bradycardia
    3. Mental confusion
    4. Distended neck veins

67. Client education regarding early signs of prostate cancer include:
    1. Difficulty in initiating urination
    2. Urinary retention and bone pain
    3. Presence of white blood cells in the urine
    4. Urinary incontinence and recurrent infections

68. A client with gastric peptic ulcer disease comes to the emergency room with palpitations, abdominal distention, pallor, and a hematocrit of 25%. The nurse would also expect the client to have:
    1. Jaundice
    2. Lightheadedness
    3. A bounding pulse
    4. An elevated serum lipase

69. An anxious client has been started on a low-dose, short-acting benzodiazepine by the physician. The nurse can expect the client to be:
    1. Euphoric and restless
    2. Calmer after the first dose
    3. Unsteady when ambulating
    4. Excessively drowsy within an hour

70. An 8-year-old girl is brought to the clinic with complaints of headaches and recurrent abdominal pain. When the nurse approaches, the child runs and hides behind her mother. After much

urging by her mother the child comes to the nurse. The nurse observes the child sucking her thumb and tugging at her hair. The nurse would most appropriately interpret that the child's behavior indicates that she is:
1. Very afraid of strangers
2. Very shy and withdrawn
3. Overly dependent on her mother
4. Exhibiting warning signs of childhood stress

71. The action by a client with an acute anxiety disorder that would indicate that the nurse has been effective in teaching how to accomplish realistic goals would be the client's:
1. Requesting to role-play a stressful situation
2. Talking about painful issues in group sessions
3. Spending less time doing negative self-evaluation
4. Breaking down problems into manageable subproblems

72. A bone marrow aspiration is to be performed on a client with leukemia. Nursing responsibilities for this procedure would include:
1. Encouraging the client to drink 2 liters of fluid the day after the test
2. Cancelling the procedure if the client's prothrombin time is 12 seconds
3. Keeping the client on nothing by mouth for 24 hours prior to the procedure
4. Applying pressure to the site for at least 5 minutes following the procedure

73. A client who is receiving filgrastim (Neupogen) following chemotherapy for cancer of the lymphatic system asks the nurse why this drug was prescribed. The nurse should explain that Neupogen:
1. Accelerates recovery of neutrophil counts following chemotherapy
2. Is a drug that is routinely recommended after a chemotherapy session
3. Stimulates the bone marrow to produce cells so anemia can be avoided
4. Has cytotoxic properties that will enhance the effects of other chemotherapeutic drugs

74. A client with small cell lung cancer who has been on chemotherapy is to receive filgrastim (Neupogen) 200 mcg subcutaneously every day for 5 days. The laboratory report that the nurse should monitor to determine efficiency of the drug is the:
1. Hemoglobin level
2. Red blood cell count
3. White blood cell count
4. Partial prothrombin time

75. The best indicator that a client with ulcerative colitis has an actual fluid deficit is:
1. A stool count of 18 episodes of diarrhea in 24 hours
2. A weight increase of 2 kg and a 24-hour output of 1000 ml
3. An admission weight of 74.3 kg and 2 days later a weight of 72 kg
4. A daily intake of 2400 ml and an output of 1600 ml, plus diarrheal stools

Comprehensive examination 2

76. A child who has leukemia is due to start chemotherapy. Before beginning any chemotherapy protocol the nurse should assess the child for:
    1. An arterial access line
    2. Fluid and electrolyte balance
    3. History of nausea and vomiting
    4. Familial allergy to methotrexate

77. When a 2-year-old child with tetrology of Fallot demonstrates cyanosis and dyspnea, it would be appropriate for the nurse to plan to position the child in the:
    1. Knee-chest position
    2. High-Fowler's position
    3. Semi-Fowler's position
    4. Trendelenburg position

78. When monitoring a male client following extracorporeal shock wave lithotripsy (ESWL) the observations that should be reported to the physician immediately would be:
    1. Dysuria on urination
    2. Intermittent hematuria
    3. Episodes of dull flank pain
    4. Persistent pain radiating to the scrotum

79. A 3-month-old infant is scheduled for surgical repair of a cleft lip. The nurse's preoperative teaching for the parents should focus on:
    1. The need for genetic counseling
    2. How they will feed the baby after surgery
    3. The types of anesthetic drugs used during surgery
    4. Their knowledge of potential surgical complications

80. Priority nursing care for for a client admitted to the hospital with the diagnosis of COPD should include:
    1. Elevating the head of the bed
    2. Providing frequent oral hygiene
    3. Encouraging a diet low in sodium
    4. Administering oxygen at 8 liters via nasal cannula

81. A newly delivered client with five children at home has deep vein thrombosis and needs to remain in the hospital on bedrest and intravenous heparin therapy. An appropriate nursing diagnosis would be:
    1. Ineffective family coping related to illness and separation
    2. Altered parenting related to added responsibilities of the new mother
    3. Altered family processes related to the prolonged absence of the mother
    4. Dysfunctional grieving related to the prolonged absence from the children

82. When a client experiences a state of acute anxiety, the endocrine glands that release hormones are the:
    1. Pancreas and thymus
    2. Thyroid and parathyroid
    3. Parathyroid and adrenal medulla
    4. Adrenal medulla and adrenal cortex

83. A psychiatric aide reports that a newly admitted female is experiencing an acute anxiety reaction. The nurse checks the client's records and notes the nursing diagnosis: Anxiety related to feelings of failure and impending doom. The nurse should first:
    1. Gently confront the client with her use of maladaptive behaviors
    2. Assist the client with managing and reducing anxiety-related symptoms
    3. Administer the prescribed PRN antianxiety medication to decrease symptoms
    4. Help the client identify the relationship between anxiety and physiologic responses

84. The extrapyramidal side effect (EPSE) that occurs as a late symptom associated with long-term use of high-dose phenothiazine drugs is:
    1. Akathisia
    2. Tardive dyskinesia
    3. Dystonia/dyskinesia
    4. Pseudo-parkinsonism

85. The nurse notices that a client scheduled for extensive surgery in the morning asks questions without waiting for the answers. The nurse diagnoses moderate anxiety related to impending surgery and sets a reduction in the level of anxiety as a goal. Goal attainment can be measured by the client's:
    1. Feeling of calmness
    2. Understanding of the surgical procedure
    3. Statement of relief of anxiety about surgery
    4. Ability to question the anesthesiologist and surgeon

86. When monitoring a client with a diagnosis of abruptio placentae the nurse is aware that the fetal finding which may be associated with this diagnosis would be:
    1. Failure to engage
    2. Late decelerations
    3. Breech presentation
    4. Variable decelerations

87. A 10-year-old with celiac disease asks the nurse, "How long will I have to remain on the special diet?" The response by the nurse that correctly reflects the length of dietary restriction is:
    1. "This diet must be maintained indefinitely."
    2. "Until you have finished your growth spurt."
    3. "Occasional dietary indiscretions are allowed."
    4. "Only until you become desensitized to gluten."

88. At the age of 4 months an infant is admitted to the hospital with a possible urinary tract infection. The data gathered from the mother that would be most significant in helping to establish this diagnosis is that the infant has:
    1. Been cranky for 2 days
    2. Recently developed a diaper rash
    3. Been having 20 to 25 slightly wet diapers a day
    4. Had a temperature between 100 and 101° F for 2 days

89. During the initial physical assessment of a newborn the nurse observes symmetric gluteal folds. The nurse should:
    1. Assess the hips for congenital dislocation
    2. Note this finding on the assessment record
    3. Palpate both thighs to ascertain Ortolani's click
    4. Notify the pediatrician immediately of the finding

90. A hematologic finding in the newborn that indicates the desired response to a vitamin K injection is an increase in the:
    1. Prothrombin level
    2. Platelet production
    3. Immunoglobulin level
    4. Hemoglobin production

91. During feeding a newborn becomes dusky with nasal flaring and intercostal and substernal retractions. Priority nursing intervention would focus on:
    1. Taking vital signs
    2. Clearing the airway
    3. Notifying the physician
    4. Administering 100% oxygen

92. At 34-weeks gestation a client is admitted to the antepartum unit with a 6 lb (2.7 kg) weight gain in one week and puffiness in her hands and ankles. A nursing diagnosis of fluid volume excess is made. Nursing interventions for this diagnosis include:
    1. Weighing weekly
    2. Maintaining bedrest
    3. Encouraging ambulation
    4. Increasing sodium intake

93. Despite hospitalization for pregnancy-induced hypertension (PIH), a client's condition seems to be worsening. Her blood pressure is now 150/100, her deep tendon reflexes are 3+, and her edema is more diffuse. The nurse understands that more aggressive pharmacologic treatment at this point is essential to prevent:
    1. Oliguria
    2. Seizures
    3. Proteinuria
    4. Respiratory arrest

94. The nurse would know that an electrocardiogram supports the diagnosis of atrial fibrillation when it demonstrates:
    1. Prolonged P-R intervals
    2. Premature atrial complexes
    3. Wide and bizarre ventricular complexes
    4. Erratic, wavy baseline between ventricular complexes

95. A 56-year-old male has had problems with dizziness, especially when turning his head to the side. Carotid artery stenosis has been diagnosed. The nurse correctly assesses the client's carotid pulses by palpating:
    1. Both carotid pulses at the same time to check for equal strength
    2. One carotid and one radial pulse at the same time to check for deficits
    3. Each carotid pulse separately to compare strength of one side to the other
    4. One carotid and the apical pulse at the same time to check for missed beats

96. A client is admitted with acute inferior myocardial infarction complicated by a right ventricular infarction. Specific to fluid administration, the nurse should monitor the client's:
    1. Heart rate
    2. Urinary output
    3. Cardiac rhythm
    4. CK isoenzymes

97. The surgeon used a client's left saphenous vein as a graft during coronary artery surgery. After surgery the client's left leg is edematous. The nurse should:
    1. Administer diuretics as ordered
    2. Request that physician order a low-salt diet
    3. Suggest the client do knee bending exercises
    4. Encourage the client to wear anti-embolic stockings

98. A client is hospitalized after falling on an icy sidewalk and fracturing the right hip. Following repair of the hip, the client has a seizure and is lying on the left side. The nurse places pillows between the client's legs to help prevent:
    1. Flexion of the hip
    2. Adduction of the hip
    3. Flexion of the knees
    4. Extension of the knees

99. The nursing care plan for an infant with bronchopulmonary dysplasia will need to include a goal on restriction of:
    1. Stimulation
    2. Fluid intake
    3. Caloric intake
    4. Ambient oxygen

100. An infant with bronchopulmonary dysplasia will need to be monitored carefully for hypothermia, hyperthermia, feeding difficulties, and:
    1. Periodic breathing
    2. Pulmonary edema
    3. Expiratory grunting
    4. Increased muscle tone

101. The nursing care plan for an infant with bronchopulmonary dysplasia (BPD) should include nursing orders relevant to:
    1. Increasing fluid intake for hydration
    2. Decreasing sensorimotor stimulation
    3. Avoiding individuals who are smoking
    4. Providing continuous gavage feedings

102. A young child's serum theophylline level is 15 mcg/ml. On the basis of this level the nurse should:
    1. Maintain seizure precautions
    2. Assess blood pressure hourly
    3. Continue with current therapy
    4. Monitor closely for cardiac dysrhythmias

103. While suctioning an unconscious client's posterior pharynx the nurse notes that the client stiffly extends, adducts, and pronates the arms and hyperextends and plantar flexes the feet. The nurse should recognize this posturing as:
    1. A sign of serious brain injury
    2. An early sign of arousal from coma
    3. The beginning of a grand mal seizure
    4. A symptom of increasing intracranial pressure

104. The assessment of a client 7 days following a heart transplant shows: T 103° F; heart rate 125; respirations 32 with dyspnea; BP 90/70; 2+ edema of ankles; and restlessness. The nurse realizes the client is probably experiencing:
    1. Pneumonia
    2. Early signs of rejection
    3. Congestive heart failure
    4. Common postoperative manifestations

105. The nurse can best demonstrate an understanding of the needs of a depressed client by:
    1. Allowing the client to set times for meals, sleep, and activities
    2. Establishing a 1-to-1 trusting, therapeutic relationship with the client
    3. Helping the client with routine hygiene so the client won't get too tired
    4. Helping the client, through the use of active listening, determine that there is nothing to be sad about

106. The nurse is aware that after detoxification from heroin, an opioid antagonist used to supplement other treatments is:
    1. Narcan
    2. Naltrexone
    3. Methadone
    4. Buprenorphine

107. The physician orders disulfiram (Antabuse) as part of a client's treatment regimen. The nurse is aware that Antabuse therapy is often used as part of an alcohol treatment program to:
    1. Modify behavior
    2. Enhance alertness
    3. Promote relaxation
    4. Lessen withdrawal symptoms

108. A client is receiving clozapine (Clozaril), an antipsychotic drug. The nurse should evaluate the client for signs of the most serious side effect, which is:
    1. Hypoglycemia
    2. Agranulocytosis
    3. Hypertensive crisis
    4. An anticholinergic reaction

109. A client whose pregnancy is progressing well asks what her blood pressure, weight, and urine have to do with her pregnancy. The best response by the nurse would be, "Although everything is fine we monitor you because:
    1. Hypertension, rapid weight gain, and/or proteinuria can indicate the beginning of a complication that can be controlled."
    2. An elevated blood pressure, rapid weight gain, and proteinuria require hospitalization before your pregnancy gets out of control."
    3. Changes in the blood pressure, weight, and urine can indicate that your blood vessels are responding negatively to the pregnancy."
    4. These are physiologic parameters for determining how well you are progressing through your pregnancy and if you will deliver on time."

110. The physician informs a pregnant client who is taking an antiepileptic drug for a poorly controlled seizure disorder that her seizures may increase during pregnancy. The nurse explains that a factor that may contribute to an exacerbation of seizures would be:
    1. Decreased estrogen levels associated with pregnancy
    2. Increased sleep and decreased stress caused by the drugs
    3. Increased respirations associated with pregnancy resulting in a mild compensatory acidosis
    4. Decreased blood levels of the antiepileptic drugs caused by the physiologic changes of pregnancy

111. An infant with a congenital heart defect is started on digoxin (Lanoxin) and furosemide (Lasix). The nursing assessment that would provide the most complete data as to the effectiveness of the Lasix in this child would be:
    1. Pulse rate
    2. Daily weight
    3. Specific gravity of urine
    4. Urinary output for 24 hours

112. The nurse is planning to care for a 10-year-old child with acute rheumatic fever. The most applicable goal for this child would be:
    1. Eliminate future episodes of the disease by vaccinating against streptococci
    2. Reduce pain to tolerable levels by administering narcotics such as meperidine
    3. Maintain physical activity by sending the child to the recreation room for bike riding three times a day
    4. Eradicate the streptococci organism in the blood and sputum cultures by administering penicillin antibiotic therapy

113. A client is admitted for the placement of a stent in the left coronary artery. In the preoperative period the nursing action that most influences reduction of anxiety in this client and the family is:
    1. Assessing the client's understanding of the seriousness of the surgery
    2. Providing preoperative teaching in terms the client and family can understand
    3. Supplying complete descriptions of the operative procedure and answering questions
    4. Explaining the cardiac rehabilitation program and reassuring the client of a quick recovery

114. A client who has had arthroscopic surgery of the knee is ready for discharge. The nurse evaluates that discharge teaching is understood when the client states:
    1. "I will notify the physician if I experience severe joint or leg pain."
    2. "I will not bend or exercise my right leg until after the 1-week checkup."
    3. "I will increase the frequency of aspirin if any joint swelling or warmth occurs."
    4. "I know increased joint pain is caused by mechanical injury and is therefore expected for 36 hours."

115. When preparing a client for percutaneous transluminal coronary angioplasty (PTCA), the nurse is aware that client education should include:
    1. Restricting oral fluids
    2. Encouraging early ambulation
    3. Discontinuing medicines following PTCA
    4. Reporting any chest discomfort following PTCA

116. When performing a postsurgical neurovascular assessment of a client with a hip fracture, the nurse notes a left dorsalis pedis pulse amplitude of +1 and a right dorsalis pedis pulse amplitude of +2. As a result of this finding the nurse would also expect to note that:
    1. The left foot is paler than the right foot
    2. The skin is cooler on the right extremity
    3. Capillary refill is quicker in the left extremity
    4. Blanching disappears more quickly on the left side

117. A client is scheduled for a bronchoscopy. The nurse, when teaching prior to the bronchoscopy, should tell the client:
    1. "You may drink liquids immediately after the procedure is done."
    2. "If you want a cigarette, you may have it after the procedure is finished."
    3. "You may be temporarily hoarse after the procedure, so do not strain your voice."
    4. "If you have excess mucus in your throat after this procedure, you may cough or clear your throat."

118. Three days following a colon resection, the client's abdomen becomes painful and boardlike. The nurse should suspect:
    1. Peritonitis
    2. Hypokalemia
    3. Paralytic ileus
    4. A bowel obstruction

119. A client is admitted to the progressive coronary care unit in congestive heart failure. The client's serum electrolytes are: BUN 18; creatinine 2.2; glucose 98; potassium 2.7; and sodium 150. The nurse would expect to administer:
    1. Bumex
    2. Glucose
    3. Aldactone
    4. Gentamycin

120. The nurse in the clinic would recognize that the statement by a client that most suggests the presence of gallbladder disease would be:
    1. "I've been gaining a lot of weight lately."
    2. "My stools are darker; sometimes they're even black."
    3. "Yesterday, when I ate a hamburger, my belly really hurt."
    4. "When I start hurting, it helps if I drink milk or have a small snack."

121. The nurse is aware that the most appropriate intravenous fluid for a client with diabetes mellitus who has dry mucous membranes, low urine output, and an abnormally high serum potassium level would be:
    1. 0.9% saline
    2. Dextrose 50%
    3. Ringers lactate
    4. Dextrose 5% and 0.45% saline

122. A 90-year-old client who has been on antibiotics for 3 days is hospitalized with lobar pneumonia. The nurse observes for the group of symptoms that would indicate complications. These symptoms would include:
    1. Occasional anorexia, fatigue, and weakness
    2. Disorientation, anorexia, and shortness of breath
    3. Increased thirst, increased urinary output, and chest pain
    4. Continuing fever, declining vital signs, and pleural effusion

123. When performing a nursing assessment of a client with a tentative diagnosis of bacterial meningitis, the nurse asks the client to flex and rotate the head. The nurse is observing for:
    1. Range of motion
    2. Signs of meningeal irritation
    3. Ability to follow spoken commands
    4. Edema of the neck and posterior portions of the head

124. In response to an elderly client's question, the nurse explains that pernicious anemia is frequently found in the older age group because the stomach mucosa fails to produce:
    1. Vitamin B_{12}
    2. Red blood cells
    3. The intrinsic factor
    4. Any extrinsic factors

125. A client with whom the nurse has been working in a one-to-one relationship for the past 3 weeks says to the nurse, "I don't want to talk to you." The nurse's best response would be:
    1. "Why don't you want to talk today?"
    2. "I'll come back when you feel like talking."
    3. "I'll just sit here quietly with you for a few minutes."
    4. "What is going on? Have I done something to anger you?"

126. A client with bone metastasis as a result of ovarian cancer comes to the clinic with signs of anorexia, nausea, polyuria, and polydipsia. Laboratory results include Hgb 18%, HCT 55%, glucose 110 mg/dl, Na 140 mEq/L, K 4.0 mEq/L, Cl 105 mEq/L, Ca 16.5 mg/dl. The nurse recognizes that these data indicate:
    1. Dehydration and hypercalcemia
    2. Overhydration and hyperkalemia
    3. Hyponatremia and hyperglycemia
    4. Hypochloremia and hypernatremia

127. The nurse stays with a mother who is having problems with breastfeeding while she feeds the baby in order to evaluate her breastfeeding technique. Indicators that the mother is breastfeeding correctly are that she holds the baby in a:
    1. Sims' position and has the mouth positioned on the nipple
    2. Football hold and has the mouth positioned to compress the nipple
    3. Trendelenburg position and has the mouth positioned over the nipple
    4. Semi-Fowler's position and has the mouth positioned to compress the areola

128. While examining their newborn following delivery, the parents say to the nurse, "We heard the Apgar scores were 8 and 10. What is an Apgar score?" The nurse tells them that the Apgar scores are used to evaluate the:
    1. Existence of a gross anamoly
    2. Presence of spontaneous breathing
    3. Baby's ability to live outside the body
    4. Baby's ability to interact with the environment

129. A client is scheduled for a Rorschach test and asks the nurse what the test is for. The nurse plans to explain to the client that the purpose of the Rorschach test is to:
    1. Graphically uncover dysfunctional family patterns
    2. Test a client's psychologic, social, and occupational functioning
    3. Reveal aspects of an individual's personality structure and emotional functioning
    4. See how the individual interprets what is happening when shown pictures of people in emotional situations

130. When a nurse responds to a client's comment by saying, "Tell me more about that." The interviewing technique being used is:
    1. Open questioning
    2. Closed questioning
    3. Probing questioning
    4. Double-barreled questioning

131. Following excision of the thyroid gland, a client is placed on thyroid hormone. The nurse knows that this medication is prescribed to:
    1. Promote hyperkinesis
    2. Increase cholinergic activity
    3. Increase the metabolic rate and calorigenesis
    4. Alter protein, fat, and carbohydrate metabolism

132. When doing preoperative counseling for a client scheduled for a radical neck resection, the nurse should include the fact that in the immediate postoperative period the client will have a:
    1. Tracheostomy, nasogastric tube to suction, and IVs
    2. Tracheostomy, nasogastric tube for feeding, and Foley catheter
    3. Gastrostomy tube to suction, chest tube to water-seal suction, and IVs
    4. Gastrectomy tube for feeding, chest tube to water-seal suction, and a Foley catheter

133. A client has sustained multiple fractures in a plane crash. The fracture that would alert the nurse to observe the client for manifestations of a fat embolus would be a fracture of the:
    1. Ribs
    2. Patella
    3. Vertebra
    4. Humerus

134. A client is admitted to the emergency room with a compression chest injury caused by the steering wheel during a motor vehicle accident. The assessment finding that should alert the nurse to a possible mediastinal shift would be:
    1. Hemoptysis
    2. Tracheal deviation
    3. Collapsed neck veins
    4. A sucking sound on inspiration

135. A client has insulin-dependent diabetes. The blood glucose indicates that regular insulin must be administered. After administering the regular insulin at 11:00 AM, the time the nurse should observe carefully for any indication of an insulin reaction would be:
    1. At bedtime
    2. Early to mid-afternoon
    3. Around the evening meal
    4. From midnight to early morning

136. A client with gastric cancer undergoes a partial gastrectomy with anastomosis to the duodenum. A nasogastric tube to low intermittent suction is in place. In the immediate postoperative period, the nurse should anticipate gastric secretions to be:
    1. Reddish
    2. Blackish
    3. Bile colored
    4. Yellowish-green

137. A client demonstrating manic behavior has been receiving lithium carbonate. The nurse evaluates the effectiveness of the drug by observing that the client exhibits a decreasing:
    1. Appetite
    2. Drowsiness
    3. Need for fluid
    4. Push of speech

138. When a client presents symptoms such as paralysis, blindness, or deafness, and no physical disorder can be identified, the nurse recognizes that the client's symptoms are probably related to:
    1. A conversion disorder
    2. A somatization disorder
    3. An obsessive-compulsive disorder
    4. An intense generalized anxiety disorder

139. Two male seniors on the high school football team are of equal height, weight, and strength. One afternoon in practice, they get into a verbal argument about a missed play. Later, as one boy is leaving the field, he picks up the large Gatorade container and dumps the ice and liquid onto the ball-boy, who is much smaller. The school nurse recognizes that this behavior is an example of:
    1. Undoing
    2. Projection
    3. Suppression
    4. Displacement

140. A mother tells the school nurse that she has withdrawn all privileges for her teenage child who has been caught skipping school. The nurse recognizes that the mother is using the behavioral concept known as:
    1. Positive punishment
    2. Negative punishment
    3. Positive reinforcement
    4. Negative reinforcement

141. When assessing an infant suspected of having Erb palsy, the nurse would expect to find:
    1. The legs positioned in abduction
    2. Stiffness of muscles in the neck and jaws
    3. Hips that are flexed and externally rotated
    4. The arm hanging limply on the affected side

142. The nurse is caring for a 6-month-old who has recently undergone a ventroperitoneal shunt revision. The child is irritable, has a high-pitched cry, and is refusing feedings. These symptoms are most likely caused by:
    1. Severe pain
    2. Stranger anxiety
    3. Shunt malfunction
    4. Formula intolerance

143. An 18-month-old is admitted to the pediatric unit for hyperpyrexia. Antipyretics and a hypothermia mattress are ordered. The nurse could best evaluate the effectiveness of interventions to reduce the fever by assessing the child's:
    1. Hydration status
    2. Skin temperature
    3. Level of consciousness every hour
    4. Rectal temperature every 30 minutes

144. Five hours after a 4-year-old is returned from the operating room following a tonsillectomy and adenoidectomy, the vital signs are: temperature 98.8° F, pulse 130, respirations 28, and blood pressure 70/40. The child is alert, but pale, and is swallowing frequently. These assessment findings are most likely caused by:
    1. Postoperative pain
    2. Postoperative dehydration
    3. A normal postoperative response
    4. A hemorrhage at the operative site

145. A client with insulin-dependent diabetes mellitus has an insulin reaction. The symptoms that the nurse would most likely expect to be present are:
    1. Warm, flushed face, nausea, and thirst
    2. Increased urinary output, hunger, and thirst
    3. Poor skin turgor, hypotension, and a blood glucose of 510
    4. Nervousness, weakness, perspiration, and mental confusion

146. An 18-year-old primigravida, 34 weeks gestation, presents in preterm labor. The client complains of the presence of a headache for the past 4 days. The nursing assessment reveals the client's blood pressure is 125/100, the urine protein is 2+, the glucose is negative, and the reflexes are 3+. The nurse understands that these are signs of:
    1. Preeclampsia
    2. HELLP syndrome
    3. Essential hypertension
    4. Pregnancy-induced hypertension

147. A 17-year-old primigravida is admitted to the maternity unit for observation for preeclampsia. Her BP is 130/78; she has gained 6 pounds in the past week; and she has a 1+ proteinuria by dipstick. After admission, priority nursing intervention would be to:
    1. Assist her into bed in a lateral position
    2. Order a high-carbohydrate, high-protein diet
    3. Monitor her for signs of a worsening condition
    4. Instruct her about increasing her fluid intake to 3000 ml daily

148. At 40 weeks a client begins labor and is placed on external fetal monitoring. Suddenly the pattern changes and the fetal heart tracing decreases at the peak of a contraction and persists for 10 seconds after the contraction. The priority nursing care should be to:
    1. Reassure the mother that this is normal as labor progresses
    2. Hang a Pitocin drip to increase contractions to speed up labor
    3. Call the physician to come and evaluate the tracing and prepare for a cesarean delivery
    4. Give a bolus of IV fluid, change the mother's position, and if pattern persists, consider the need for getting an order for oxygen

149. Clients with AIDS may be infected by *Pneumocystis carinii*, which is a rare, parasitic, protozoan lung infection. The nurse should be aware that associated symptoms include:
    1. Cyanosis and weight loss
    2. High fever and air hunger
    3. Dyspnea and bradycardia
    4. Nonproductive cough and edema

150. A 55-year-old client is admitted with an acute episode of diverticulitis. The client's symptom that the nurse should promptly report to the physician would be:
    1. Midabdominal pain radiating to the back
    2. Nausea and vomiting periodically for several hours
    3. Abdominal rigidity with pain in the left lower quadrant
    4. Elimination pattern of constipation alternating with diarrhea

Comprehensive examination 3

151. A client who has just had a left modified radical mastectomy has two drainage tubes attached to a Y connector and a portable wound suction. Six hours later the nurse notices that there is 120 ml of drainage, the BP is 90/60, the pulse is 100, and the dressing is dry and intact. The nurse concludes that this is:
    1. A normal amount of drainage and observation will be continued every 4 hours
    2. Normal because the dressing is dry and intact and observation will be continued every hour
    3. Less than the expected drainage, the physician should be notified, and observation of the client continued
    4. More than the expected drainage, the physician should be notified, and observation of the client continued hourly

152. A client has a resection of an aortic aneurysm with placement of a Dacron graft. Postoperatively the client should be positioned in the:
    1. Supine position
    2. Trendelenberg position
    3. Left side-lying position with the knees flexed
    4. High-Fowler's position with the bed gatched at the knees

153. When preparing to transfuse a child with a unit of packed red cells, the nurse must be aware that the IV solution that is compatible with blood components is:
    1. 5% dextrose
    2. Normal saline
    3. Lactated Ringer's
    4. Normal saline and 5% dextrose

154. The nurse explains to a parent that the anemia in sickle cell disease is caused by:
    1. Increased blood viscosity
    2. Increased red cell destruction
    3. Increased white cell production
    4. Decreased red blood cell precursors

155. A 5-year-old child with leukemia is receiving a second unit of packed red blood cells. The first unit was transfused without any problems but soon after the start of the second unit, the child develops an expiratory wheeze. The priority nursing action is to:
    1. Speak calmly to help the child relax
    2. Stop the transfusion and keep the vein open
    3. Slow the rate of transfusion and monitor the child's breathing
    4. Consult with the physician about these early symptoms of asthma

156. An infant with a cleft lip and palate begins to choke while feeding. The nurse should give priority to:
    1. Asking another nurse to call a code
    2. Setting up a suction unit for rapid intervention
    3. Turning the infant to the side to let the mouth drain
    4. Watching the cardiac monitor for signs of apnea or bradycardia

157. A 17-year-old who was inhaling gasoline fumes sustained full-thickness burns over 40% of the body when the gasoline accidentally ignited. Initial nursing care should be based on the assessment of the client's:
    1. Burn status
    2. Level of addiction
    3. Fluid volume status
    4. Respiratory involvement

158. Following surgery, a client has an indwelling urinary catheter attached to a collection bag. The nurse empties the collection bag at 9:00 AM. At the change of shift at 3:00 PM the collection bag contains 100 ml of urine. The system has no obstructions to urinary flow. The nurse's most appropriate initial response would be to:
    1. Elevate the head of the client's bed
    2. Start giving the client 8 ounces of oral fluid per hour
    3. Check circulation and take the vital signs of the client
    4. Continue monitoring because this is an expected finding

159. Assumptions and roles of nurse therapists vary depending on the theoretical framework they elect or select to follow. When the nurse contracts with the client for specific behavioral changes, such as habit control, the model used would be the:
    1. Gestalt model
    2. Behaviorist model
    3. Crisis intervention model
    4. Nondirective counseling model

160. The nurse, aware of Piaget's theory of cognitive development, recognizes that the essential task for the school-age child (7 to 11 years of age) is to learn:
    1. How to reason in a logical manner
    2. To think in terms of mental images
    3. About the self and the environment
    4. To master information processing and problem solving

161. The nurse could best establish an initial baseline assessment of a newly admitted psychiatric client from the:
    1. Client
    2. Spouse or family
    3. History and physical
    4. Mental status examination

162. The verbalization offered by a client that would be most characteristic of the diagnosis of borderline personality disorder, acting-out behavior, would be:
    1. "I just heard the voices telling me to scratch my face."
    2. "I feel so ashamed. I just don't know what came over me."
    3. "I just felt so overwhelmed and hopeless about anything changing in my life."
    4. "If the other nurse had just let me go on my lobby privileges nothing would have happened."

163. After a splenectomy, the nurse should recognize an indication of an early postoperative complication if the client has:
    1. Decrease in appetite or thirst
    2. Hiccoughs and/or increased temperature
    3. Upper abdominal pain and incisional tenderness
    4. Increased gastric motility and increased urinary output

164. The nurse is aware that during pregnancy, the glomerular filtration rate:
    1. Is unaffected by gestation
    2. Decreases below prepregnant levels
    3. Increases significantly above prepregnant levels
    4. Changes only when pathologic conditions develop

165. The nursery nurse understands that when the eyes of a newborn are treated by instilling a prophylactic antimicrobial ophthalmic ointment, it is done to protect the infant against:
    1. Syphilis
    2. Trichomoniasis
    3. TORCH organisms
    4. Gonorrhea or chlamydia infections

166. A client is receiving cyclophosphamide (Cytoxan) and doxorubicin hydrochloride (Adriamycin) on an outpatient basis. Prior to chemotherapy administration the priority assessment by the nurse should be:
    1. Electrolyte balance
    2. Neurologic function
    3. Hematopoietic activity
    4. Musculoskeletal integrity

167. The nurse may need to teach the client with a spinal cord injury how to perform urinary catheterization. The method commonly used for home urinary management involves:
    1. Intermittent method using clean technique
    2. Intermittent method using sterile technique
    3. Continuous drainage using clean technique
    4. Continuous drainage using sterile technique

168. Blood and urine samples are sent to the laboratory for a client who has had a spinal cord injury. The results show: blood RBCs 3,500,000; blood WBCs 5,000; urine RBCs 1 to 2; and urine WBCs 11,000. After reviewing these results, the nurse should be alert for signs of:
    1. Anemia
    2. Septicemia
    3. Gross hematuria
    4. Urinary tract infection

169. The nurse plans bladder retraining for a client using the Credé maneuver. This technique involves:
    1. Using a special Credé urinary catheter on a fixed time schedule
    2. Pressing down on the bladder with a fisted hand using a rolling motion
    3. Slowly inserting a finger into the rectum until the perineal muscles relax
    4. Holding one's breath and bearing down as if attempting a bowel movement

170. The nurse, aware that Parkinson's disease is a complex clinical syndrome with alterations in motor function, assesses a client with this diagnosis for:
    1. Seizures and coma
    2. Tremors and rigidity
    3. Spasticity and rigidity
    4. Paraesthesia and paralysis

171. When answering a client's questions about the Mantoux test for tuberculosis, the nurse should base the response on the fact that the:
    1. Area of erythema is measured in 3 days and determines if tuberculosis is present
    2. Skin test does not differentiate between active and dormant tuberculosis infection
    3. Presence of a wheal at the site of injection in 2 days indicates the presence of tuberculosis
    4. Test stimulates an erythemal response in some clients and a second test may be done in 3 months

172. During the assessment of an 18-year-old with a cerebral glioma, the nurse notes left-sided weakness and a decreased response of the left pupil. The most appropriate nursing diagnosis would be:
    1. Anxiety related to impending surgery for glioma
    2. Altered vision related to blindness caused by tumor
    3. Dressing/grooming self-care deficit related to motor impairment
    4. Altered nutrition: less than body requirements, related to cachexia caused by the tumor

173. Following an exploratory laparotomy and intestinal resection, a client returns from surgery with a large abdominal dressing and two negative pressure drains. On the initial assessment, the nurse notices the abdominal dressing is damp. The nurse should:
    1. Estimate the amount of wound drainage
    2. Remove the dressing to assess the wound
    3. Change the dressing using sterile technique
    4. Place a sterile dressing over the existing one

174. The physician orders an indwelling urinary catheter for a client who has received abdominal injuries in a train accident. While preparing for the catheterization, the nurse notices blood at the urethral meatus. The nurse should:
    1. Gently irrigate the urethra with sterile saline or water
    2. Insert the catheter and hyperinflate the catheter balloon
    3. Hemoccult the urethral discharge before catheterization
    4. Postpone catheterization and notify the physician of the findings

175. The nurse is aware of the importance of preventing an air embolism during the initial insertion of a central venous line or later during tubing changes. The most effective nursing action to prevent this complication during the procedure would be to:
    1. Place the client in a low-Fowler's position
    2. Have the client perform the Valsalva maneuver
    3. Have the client assume a high-Fowler's position
    4. Ask the client to turn the head to the opposite side

176. The primary consideration when caring for a child with sickle cell anemia is to:
    1. Supply diversional activities
    2. Keep the child well-hydrated
    3. Provide supplemental oxygen
    4. Perform passive range of motion to painful joints

177. A 14-year-old has had arthroscopic surgery to the knee following a gymnastic accident. When instructing the mother regarding care after discharge from ambulatory surgery, the nurse should include the fact that the teenager:
    1. Should have the dressing changed every 6 hours
    2. May have some light pink drainage on the knee dressing
    3. Should start exercising the knee later on in the afternoon
    4. May return to school the next day if there is no drowsiness

178. A 15-month-old is admitted to the pediatric unit. The assessment that should most concern the nurse would be the:
    1. Child weighing 15.4 lb (7 kg)
    2. Child's failure to smile frequently
    3. Child's inability to walk unassisted
    4. Child crying when approached by hospital staff

179. The most effective nursing action to help new parents bond with their newborn who has a cleft lip and palate would be:
    1. Reassuring the parents of the success of plastic surgery
    2. Identifying the roles of the cleft lip/palate team to the couple
    3. Recommending that the parents receive emotional counseling
    4. Emphasizing to the couple the positive aspects of the child's appearance

180. A neonate, born with a sac over the lower lumbar region, is transported to the neonatal intensive care unit for diagnosis and treatment. A nursing assessment that would be especially important to assist in the diagnosis would be:
    1. Length
    2. Blood glucose
    3. Specific gravity
    4. Head circumference

181. The care plan for a client with an abruptio placentae, who has just been admitted to the labor room suite, will most likely include the nursing diagnosis:
    1. Pain related to blood trapped behind placenta
    2. Decreased cardiac output related to blood loss
    3. Family coping: potential for growth related to loss
    4. Fear related to concern over personal and fetal safety

182. A client with an amniotic fluid embolus is in danger of developing an:
    1. Atonic uterus
    2. Underlying pneumonia
    3. Inadequate placental expulsion
    4. Occlusion of the pulmonary capillaries

183. Knowing the toxic effects of oral contraceptives, the nurse instructs a client to report immediately the presence of:
    1. Angina
    2. Chloasma
    3. Metrorrhagia
    4. Dysmenorrhea

184. An assessment of a neonate reveals the following characteristics: LGA (macrosomic); color ruddy; plethoric; rounded face, and prominent abdomen. These assessments indicate that this may be an infant who:
    1. Is postterm
    2. Has Down syndrome
    3. Has erythroblastosis fetalis
    4. Is born to an insulin-dependent diabetic mother

185. A client arrives alone at the labor room suite in active labor. She has had no prenatal care and is vague about the time of conception. During the initial history taking the client is quite jumpy, has a running nose, and does a good deal of sniffing. An additional assessment that would contribute to the nurse's suspicion that the client is a drug abuser would be:
    1. A low pain tolerance
    2. A dirty and unkempt appearance
    3. The lack of a support person during labor
    4. The presence of controlled behavior during labor

186. A client who has a history of intermittent hypertension of 200 to 260 systolic and 170 to 180 diastolic is suspected of having pheochromocytoma. A urine test for vanillylmandelic acid (VMA) is ordered. The nurse could best explain this test to the client by stating, "You:
    1. Must collect all urine for 24 hours and it will be tested for products resulting from adrenal activity."
    2. Must receive an injection of dye, and your urine will be saved to measure the speed of the dye elimination."
    3. Will be given a drug, and the response of your body will be evaluated by monitoring your blood pressure and heart rate."
    4. Will be given an insulin and glucose solution, and the sugar in your urine and blood will be compared at set time intervals."

187. The husband of a client who has bacterial meningitis is concerned that the room has been darkened by closing the blinds and turning down the lights. The nurse explains that the major reason for this nursing action is to:
    1. Promote rest and relaxation to facilitate healing
    2. Decrease anxiety by facilitating a calm atmosphere
    3. Reduce sensory stimulation to decrease chance of seizure activity
    4. Prevent further deterioration in the mental status by decreasing eye movement

188. A client who has smoked for 40 years was diagnosed with chronic obstructive pulmonary disease several years ago. The client is admitted to the hospital with dyspnea, cyanosis, and wheezing. The nursing care for this client should include:
   1. Restricting fluids
   2. Providing for planned rest periods
   3. Placing in the Trendelenburg position
   4. Administering high amounts of oxygen

189. An expected outcome for a client with pneumonia is: "The airway will be free of secretions." To help assure this outcome the nurse should:
   1. Monitor oxyhemoglobin saturation by oximetry
   2. Assess color of skin, lips, and nail beds for cyanosis
   3. Question an order for a cough suppressant medication
   4. Reduce overtiring by pacing care to ensure oxygen delivery to tissues

190. An 88-year-old client is an active resident in a retirement village where a one-bedroom apartment is shared with a sibling. The client has bilateral cataracts and can only detect degrees of light. An inpatient, left-eye, lens removal and transplant is planned. Considering the history and physical status, the best room in which to place this client is a:
   1. Private room next to the nursing station
   2. Room situated away from traffic and activity
   3. Negative pressure room on contact isolation
   4. Semi-private room with an alert person of the same age

191. Following a partial thyroidectomy, the manifestations that would most likely suggest to the nurse that the client was having a thyroid crisis would be:
   1. Facial numbness and twitching
   2. High body temperature and tachycardia
   3. Subnormal blood pressure and syncope
   4. Extreme sedation with frequent yawning

192. The nurse is aware that a child who fails to master Erikson's developmental task of autonomy vs. shame and doubt may demonstrate:
   1. Feelings of inferiority
   2. A chronic mistrust of others
   3. A sense of guilt and insecurity
   4. Difficulty with interpersonal relationships

193. A client in the mental health clinic tells the nurse, "During the last 10 years I've been promoted 4 times, and now I am laid off and very concerned about my future." In order to convey empathy and show understanding, the nurse's best response would be:
   1. "You wonder how this could happen to you?"
   2. "That must be a terrible disappointment to you."
   3. "What do you think went wrong that this happened?"
   4. "Sure you are. But I am sure everything will be all right."

194. The nurse should teach the client and client's family that the antipsychotic drug clozapine (Clozaril) has as its most serious side effect:
   1. Seizures
   2. Sedation
   3. Hypotension
   4. Agranulocytosis

195. The nurse is aware that children with fears about being in school usually demonstrate:
   1. The need to excel
   2. Fears of social situations
   3. A lack of trust in authority figures
   4. A need to be in control of situations

196. A client is admitted with cognitive dysfunction caused by prolonged exposure to toxic industrial wastes. The type of behavior that the nurse would expect this client to exhibit would include:
   1. Sleeping 10 hours or more each night
   2. Irritability to external stimuli on the unit
   3. Difficulty in expressing ideas and needs
   4. Inability to eat without experiencing nausea

197. The plan of care to meet a disturbed male client's hygiene needs during his initial attempts at self-care should include:
   1. Limiting staff involvement in his care
   2. Providing an electric razor for shaving
   3. Administering medication prior to morning care
   4. Bathing him, but permitting him to dress himself

198. A child who is HIV positive is receiving didanosine (ddl; Videx) therapy. The nurse would suspect an adverse reaction to this medication if the child develops:

1. Muscle wasting
2. Growth retardation
3. A learning disability
4. A peripheral neuropathy

199. The nurse is able to evaluate that the parents understand the long-term care for a child who has had a cleft palate repair when they state:
    1. "Soft foods are best for our child."
    2. "We'll be sure to watch for ear infections."
    3. "We have to keep our child from laughing."
    4. "Now speech therapy will not be necessary."

200. The nurse is assessing an adolescent who is experiencing a sickle cell crisis (pain episode). The nurse would best be able to achieve the goal of relieving the pain by:
    1. Giving an oral analgesic per physician's orders
    2. Providing comfort measures such as a backrub
    3. Giving morphine sulfate once per day per physician's orders
    4. Administering continuous IV drip analgesia per physician's orders

201. The nurse obtains a history from a mother whose 18-month-old daughter is suspected of having lead poisoning. The statement in the child's history that would be characteristic of lead poisoning is "My daughter:
    1. Has been having temper tantrums."
    2. Seems to be hungry all the time lately."
    3. Cannot yet walk downstairs without help."
    4. Used to eat from a spoon without spilling, but she can't anymore."

202. A nurse in a family planning clinic has completed home care instructions for a client who has had a vasectomy. The client's statement that suggests the nurse's instructions have been misunderstood would be:
    1. "I'll still be able to have an orgasm and ejaculate even after the procedure."
    2. "It's a relief to know that this won't affect sensation and having an erection."
    3. "There has been some success in restoring a man's fertility after a vasectomy."
    4. "Now that this is done, we don't need to be concerned about birth control anymore."

203. A client is admitted to the hospital with a bleeding gastric ulcer. During the assessment the nurse would expect the client to describe the pain as:
    1. Intermittent and colicky in the flank area
    2. Dull, aching, and radiating to the left side
    3. A gnawing sensation that is eased after eating
    4. A generalized discomfort that is worse with movement

204. A client with lung cancer is receiving chemotherapy and is having episodes of nausea and vomiting. The client is receiving prochlorperazine (Compazine) before meals. One hour after eating, the client is found sedated with a respiratory rate of 8 and a pulse oximetry of 85%. The nurse should first:
    1. Arouse the client to take several deep breaths
    2. Report the observation to the client's physician
    3. Adjust the pulse oximetry lead placement and re-evaluate
    4. Place the client on humidified oxygen by nasal cannula or mask

205. The birth record of a newly delivered infant reveals that the mother's membranes ruptured 36 hours prior to delivery and low forceps were required for delivery. The infant is assessed as a fullterm infant with an Apgar of 8/9. Based on these findings, nursing interventions for the infant should be planned to include:
    1. Enriching the environment with 40% oxygen to improve depressed Apgars
    2. Providing routine nursery care, because all findings are within normal limits
    3. Observing for possible infection as a result of prolonged premature rupture of the membranes
    4. Positioning with the head slightly elevated to decrease potential cerebral damage from the use of forceps

206. When interpreting the laboratory results of a prenatal client, the nurse understands that the finding that would require follow-up care is:
    1. Rubella titer 1:8
    2. WBC 10,500 mm^3
    3. VDRL-nonreactive
    4. Hemoglobin 12.5 g

207. A client has cataract surgery of the right eye late in the afternoon. The client is found sleeping on the right side with the head of the bed slightly elevated. At this time it would be most therapeutic for the nurse to:
    1. Allow the client to sleep undisturbed
    2. Gently repositon the client to the back
    3. Awaken the client and assess the right eye
    4. Lower the head of the bed to keep the client flat

208. Three days before bowel surgery the surgeon orders a clear liquid diet, neomycin, and GoLYTELY. The nurse should explain to the client that these measures are used to:
    1. Prevent dehydration before surgery
    2. Prevent bowel obstruction before surgery
    3. Decrease the risk of postoperative sepsis
    4. Decrease the amount of ileal drainage after surgery

209. A 55-year-old woman is admitted for a left modified radical mastectomy. The nurse plans that a priority outcome on the day of surgery will be, "The client will:
    1. Demonstrate wound care and discuss how to care for the incision."
    2. Experience no unnecessary discomfort and maintain circulating fluid volume."
    3. Maintain circulating fluid volume and discuss the impact of the loss of her breast."
    4. Demonstrate left shoulder exercises twice and experience no unnecessary discomfort."

210. A client, at 32-weeks gestation, calls the prenatal clinic to report that she is experiencing contractions. The nurse suspects this client is in preterm labor because the contractions are occurring:
    1. Every 10 minutes and lasting 30 seconds
    2. Every 15 minutes and lasting 45 seconds
    3. Every 20 minutes and lasting 30 seconds
    4. Every 30 minutes and lasting 45 seconds

211. A client who is experiencing severe pain in the right leg on activity is being prepared for a percutaneous transluminal angioplasty. The nurse reinforces the information provided by the physician and answers questions. The nurse knows the information has been understood when the client states:
    1. "I will be able to walk in my room after the doctor finishes."
    2. "There is a chance that I could bleed or need more surgery."
    3. "A friend of mine had this done and he went home the same day."
    4. "I will be asleep during the procedure and shouldn't have problems."

212. A client with insulin-dependent diabetes mellitus has an insulin reaction and is admitted unconscious to the hospital. The order for this client that the nurse should question is:
    1. Glucagon 1 mg IM
    2. 50% dextrose 50 ml IV
    3. Humulin R insulin 10 units IV
    4. Epinephrine 1:1000 0.5 ml IM

213. A client with pernicious anemia is to receive vitamin B_{12} intramuscularly. It is most important that the nurse plans to emphasize to the client that this therapy must be:
    1. Stopped when symptoms disappear
    2. Continued for the rest of the client's life
    3. Administered every 6 months by the visiting nurse
    4. Taken by mouth once the maintenance dose is determined

214. Following surgery, in the postanesthesia recovery room, a client is placed on patient controlled analgesia (PCA). On the second postoperative day the client tells the nurse that the pump is not relieving the pain. The nurse's initial response should be to:
    1. Gently flush the IV to ensure it is patent
    2. Determine the client's understanding of the PCA
    3. Engage the PCA and administer a dose to the client
    4. Inform the physician that the prescribed dose is not sufficient

215. A client's tracheostomy needs suctioning. The best procedure for the nurse to follow is to:
    1. Pour sterile water into the suction kit, put on clean gloves, pick up the suction catheter, then turn on the suction
    2. Pour sterile normal saline into the suction kit, pick up suction catheter with ungloved hand and connect to suction source, then turn on suction

3. Turn on the suction, pour sterile water into the suction kit, pick up the sterile catheter with the gloved hand, then connect it to the suction source
4. Turn on the suction, pour sterile normal saline into the suction kit, put on sterile gloves, pick up the suction catheter with gloved hand, then connect to suction source

216. The nurse is able to evaluate the parents' understanding of their adolescent's persistent vegetative state following a severe head injury by:
    1. Having a private discussion with the parents
    2. Observing the frequency and length of parental visits
    3. Asking the parents to review the physiologic progress
    4. Referring the parents to a psychologist and reviewing the report

217. The physician prescribes the antidepressant drug imipramine (Tofranil) for a depressed client. The nurse should be aware that Tofranil, like other antidepressant medications, may:
    1. Mask the symptoms of a suicide
    2. Cause liver damage and cerebral hemorrhage
    3. Have little effect unless it is administered with another drug
    4. Produce a mood elevation only with exogenous depression

218. A client with a long history of schizophrenia is readmitted after forgetting to take the tranquilizers that have been prescribed. The client has no family or friends, lacks social skills, and has poor impulse control. A priority nursing diagnosis for this client at this time would be:
    1. Hopelessness related to feelings of isolation
    2. Risk for injury related to poor impulse control
    3. Social isolation related to the lack of social skills
    4. Noncompliance with treatment related to not remembering to take medication

219. The behavior that would indicate a positive treatment outcome in a female client admitted for recurrent panic attacks would be that the client:
    1. Spends the evenings quietly in her room
    2. Asks for her prn medication only twice a day
    3. Suggests a movie outing for the therapy group
    4. Sits on the edge of her seat during group therapy sessions

220. The physician prescribes danazol (Danocrine) for treatment of endometriosis. The nurse is aware that this medication is an effective treatment because it:
    1. Stimulates ovarian function
    2. Triggers a marked LH surge
    3. Stimulates estrogen secretion
    4. Decreases FSH and LH secretion

221. While doing shallow breathing during the transition stage of labor, a client experiences tingling and numbness of her fingertips. The nurse suggests that she breathe into:
    1. A paper bag
    2. An oxygen mask
    3. An incentive spirometer
    4. A compressed air mask

222. The nurse is teaching a client with dementia to participate in self-care. The nurse is aware that the best way to teach this client would be to:
    1. Write down all information
    2. Introduce new material daily
    3. Ask questions to obtain feedback
    4. Use simple diagrams and drawings

223. While mixing a parenteral dose of a chemotherapy drug for a child with leukemia, some of the drug splashes on the nurse's arm. The nurse's first action should be to:
    1. Rinse the area with water and notify the physician
    2. Wash off the medication with soap and resume work
    3. Simply wipe off the fluid and report the loss of the drug
    4. Absorb the fluid by patting it with gauze before wiping it off

224. The nursing diagnosis with the highest priority for a child with idiopathic thrombocytopenic purpura (ITP) is:
    1. Pain related to rash
    2. Risk for infection related to rash
    3. Risk for injury related to low platelet count
    4. Altered breathing pattern related to low pO_2

225. A mother calls the clinic nurse to ask what to do for her toddler's skin reaction and itching following exposure to poison ivy. The nurse should plan the health teaching to focus on:
1. Treating the blisters like burns
2. Identification of the poison ivy plant
3. Providing cool compresses and topical corticosteroids
4. Use of detergent soaps to wash off the poison ivy chemical

Comprehensive examination 4

226. An eighth grader is sent to the school nurse by a teacher who notices slash marks on both wrists. As part of the initial assessment, it would be most therapeutic for the nurse to ask:
    1. "Why did you do this?"
    2. "What happened to your wrists?"
    3. "It looks like you tried to kill yourself."
    4. "What did you hope to accomplish by doing this?"

227. A young teenager is admitted after an unsuccessful suicide attempt. A nursing diagnosis of ineffective individual coping is formulated. Based on this diagnosis, an important early nursing intervention should focus on:
    1. Development of insight
    2. Identification of a support system
    3. Improvement of peer relationships
    4. Enhancement of family relationships

228. An adolescent's Monospot is positive for infectious mononucleosis. The nurse should plan the adolescent's nursing care to focus on:
    1. Resuming daily activities
    2. Providing comfort measures
    3. Providing a low carbohydrate diet
    4. Establishing a history of social contacts

229. The nurse can accurately evaluate that a mother understands the immunization process for hepatitis B for her 1-month-old infant when the mother states:
    1. "My baby still needs one more hepatitis B immunization."
    2. "My baby will get a hepatitis B shot each time the polio vaccine is given."
    3. "My baby will be scheduled for the next hepatitis B shot at 2 years of age."
    4. "I'll bring the baby back to the clinic for the next hepatitis B dose in 3 months."

230. Because of frequent vomiting, babies with pyloric stenosis become dehydrated and should be assessed for:
    1. Dilute urine
    2. Weight loss
    3. Bulging fontanels
    4. Decreased hemoglobin

231. A newly admitted 2-day-old infant has a high-pitched cry and tremors. The infant is irritable and the urine has tested positive for cocaine. The nurse's initial care for this infant would be to:
    1. Place the infant on peripheral IV fluids
    2. Obtain a medication order for phenobarbital
    3. Contact the state's child protection services
    4. Provide supportive care by holding the infant

232. A 3-year-old is brought to the emergency service after ingesting 25 tablets of children's acetaminophen while at home with a baby sitter. The nurse is to give a lavage of activated charcoal followed by Mucomyst (*N*-acetylcysteine) via a nasogastric tube. The initial nursing intervention should be focused on:
    1. Calming the child
    2. Informing the parents
    3. Placing the nasogastric tube correctly
    4. Determining the time of the child's last meal

233. The physician's order for a client reads, "Haloperidol (Haldol) po 2 mg bid." The nurse is aware that the client should be assessed for:
    1. Extreme nausea and vomiting
    2. Muscular rigidity and drooling
    3. Excessive thirst and diaphoresis
    4. Jaundice and elevated blood pressure

234. When teaching about delusions, the nurse could best describe a delusion as a:
    1. Lack of insight
    2. Absence of trust
    3. Promise not kept
    4. Protection of the mind

235. The nurse is aware that respiratory distress syndrome is associated with lung maturity in the neonate. During pregnancy, evidence of fetal lung maturity may be assessed by:
    1. An oxytocic challenge test
    2. Analysis of the amniotic fluid
    3. A fetal heart rate of 128 to 168 beats per minute
    4. Ultrasound assessment of fetal respiratory movement

236. A preterm infant is placed in an Isolette with oxygen. The nurse is aware that it is important to monitor the pO_2 every hour when administering oxygen to the preterm infant because high oxygen levels predispose the infant to the development of:
    1. Patent ductus arteriosus
    2. Retinopathy of prematurity
    3. Respiratory distress syndrome
    4. Neonatal necrotizing enterocolitis

237. Immediately postpartum in the recovery room, a client who has just had a cesarean delivery needs to be assessed. This would be done by:
    1. Palpating her fundus and observing her lochia as in every delivery
    2. Observing her lochia but not palpating the fundus because of the method of delivery
    3. Palpating her fundus but realizing there will be no lochia because of the method of delivery
    4. Asking the client to palpate her own fundus to decrease the discomfort caused by the nurse's hands

238. The drug the nurse will keep at the bedside to counteract the toxic effects of magnesium sulfate therapy in clients with preeclampsia is:
    1. Ferrous sulfate
    2. Calcium gluconate
    3. Phenobarbital sodium
    4. Epinephrine hydrochloride

239. A client with chronic undifferentiated schizophrenia, living in a group home, is continually readmitted to the mental health unit because of failure to take the prescribed medications. The client states, "I want to stay out and although I try not to, I forget to take my pills." The nurse could best help the client by:
    1. Providing money for the medications when the client is discharged
    2. Requesting the client's physician to order a long-acting tranquilizer for the client
    3. Teaching the client the importance of taking the medication as prescribed
    4. Setting up a system with the client to check off medication times for each dose each day

240. A 7-year-old boy with a history of autism is admitted for emergency surgery. The nurse assesses that the child is emotionally distant from those around him and formulates a goal of improved communication. To attain this goal, the nurse should:
    1. Introduce the child to several children on the unit
    2. Visit the child for short intervals as frequently as possible
    3. Take the child to the playroom to be with the other children
    4. Request that staff members visit the child as frequently as possible

241. Based on an assessment leading to the nursing diagnosis of defensive coping, an appropriate outcome for the client would be that the client:
    1. Recognizes own mistrust and use of projective thinking
    2. Makes requests clearly and openly without hidden messages
    3. Demonstrates calm, consistent emotions when interacting with others
    4. Significantly reduces the use of manipulative behavior as a means of meeting needs

242. The nurse expects that fluid and electrolyte management for the first 72 hours following radical neck dissection will include:
    1. Clear liquid diet, IVs and I & O
    2. NPO, IV fluids and nasogastric tube to suction
    3. Nasogastric feedings at 50 ml/hour after the first 12 hours
    4. Clear fluid as soon as gag reflex returns, progressing to soft diet

243. Nursing intervention to promote airway clearance in the immediate postoperative period following a radical neck dissection would include positioning the client:
    1. Prone, and assessing vital signs q4hr
    2. With the head of bed elevated 30°, and vital signs qid
    3. Supine and assessing for dyspnea, cyanosis, and stridor q2hr
    4. With the head of bed elevated 45°, and assessing for dyspnea, cyanosis, and stridor q1hr

244. To prevent nutritional problems caused by immobility from occurring in the client who is in traction the nurse should provide the client with:
    1. Small, frequent high-fiber meals
    2. High caloric, high-protein meals
    3. Frequent servings of high-carbohydrate foods
    4. Large amounts of high-fat, high-vitamin C foods

245. A 12-year-old female with cystic fibrosis is admitted with severe bronchopneumonia. Nursing care besides management of the respiratory problems includes:
    1. Avoidance of dietary salt and fats
    2. Replacement of digestive enzymes
    3. Return to a physical exercise program
    4. Maintenance in a flat or low Fowler's position

246. Before discharge, the nurse evaluates a client's understanding of self-care of an ileostomy. The nurse would know that the teaching was effective when the client states, "I will:
   1. Irrigate the stoma after breakfast."
   2. Drink at least 2 to 3 liters of fluid daily."
   3. Avoid getting the stoma wet when bathing."
   4. Order a year's supply of ostomy equipment."

247. A 5-year-old child is admitted with acute glomerulonephritis. When taking the child's history, the nurse asks the parents if their:
   1. Child's clothes fit much more tightly lately
   2. Child has had a recent significant weight loss
   3. Child was drinking more fluids and urinating more often
   4. Child had a streptococcal infection in the past 10 to 14 days

248. A client with congestive heart failure says to the nurse, "I just can't seem to do anything anymore without getting out of breath." The nurse understands that this dyspnea is caused by the:
   1. Accumulation of fluid in the alveolar spaces
   2. Compression of lung tissue by a dilated heart
   3. Obstruction of the bronchi by mucus secretions
   4. Restriction of respiratory movement by chest pain

249. Culture and sensitivity tests on the cerebrospinal fluid of a client confirm a diagnosis of bacterial meningitis. The physician orders intravenous penicillin G to be administered every 8 hours. The client asks when isolation can be discontinued. The best reply by the nurse would be:
   1. "You will be in an isolation room until you are discharged."
   2. "At least one more day, or until your cultures are negative."
   3. "As soon as your temperature remains normal for 24 hours."
   4. "As soon as antibiotic therapy is begun, isolation restrictions will stop."

250. A client with Graves disease has medication ordered to control the symptoms of the disorder. One of the drugs ordered is propranolol (Inderal). When monitoring this client, the symptom that the nurse should report to the physician would be:
   1. Diaphoresis
   2. Bradycardia
   3. Hypertension
   4. Exophthalmos

251. A client with Graves disease is to have I^{131} therapy. It is most important that the nurse include in directions to the client that:
   1. There should be no discomfort in the neck area
   2. The client will be admitted to the hospital for the procedure
   3. At least 2000 to 3000 ml of fluid should be consumed daily for 2 to 3 days
   4. Contact with a pregnant sister and an infant daughter may be immediately resumed

252. A client has been diagnosed with insulin-dependent diabetes mellitus. When teaching the client about the disease, the nurse includes the importance of exercise to help control the serum glucose level. The response by the client that best indicates an understanding of this instruction would be:
   1. "I may exercise with a blood glucose above 350 to lower it."
   2. "I will eat 1 hour before exercising at my insulin's peak time."
   3. "I will exercise before lunch and take regular insulin at 8:00 AM."
   4. "High-impact jumping aerobics can be helpful in lowering my blood glucose."

253. A client's apical heart rate drops to 50 beats/min following cardiac surgery and an external temporary pacemaker is initiated at a demand (synchronous) rate of 70 beats/min. The next day the nurse assesses the client and finds the following: BP 120/70, apical heart rate 85 beats/min, urine output 100 ml for 2 hours, and a serum potassium level of 4.2 mEq/L. In response to these assessment findings the nurse should:
   1. Chart the findings
   2. Call the physician
   3. Start a potassium drip
   4. Cough and deep breathe the client

254. Four days after an abdominal-perineal resection a client calls the nurse and states, "It feels like something popped." The perineal dressing is dry and intact but the abdominal dressing is saturated with serosanguinous drainage. When

assessing the wound, the nurse sees the intestines exposed. The nurse should take the client's vital signs, call the surgeon, and cover the abdominal wound with a:
1. Clean dry dressing
2. Sterile pressure dressing
3. Povidone iodine dressing
4. Sterile moist saline dressing

255. On the first postoperative day following cataract surgery of the left eye, a client reports to the nurse that the left eye "aches a little bit." The nurse should first:
1. Call the physician to report the client's eye pain
2. Instruct the client to gently "blink and roll" the eyes
3. Remove the client's eye dressing and assess the eye for bleeding
4. Administer the prescribed analgesic and assess the effect in 1 hour

256. A client delivers a baby boy in the 40th week. The baby has a heel stick test done for PKU. The nurse explains to the mother that this test is done to:
1. Ascertain the baby's bilirubin level
2. Rule out hidden neurologic defects
3. Detect an inborn error of metabolism
4. Determine the level of pancreatic enzymes

257. During an acute exacerbation of rheumatoid arthritis the most appropriate nursing intervention for a client would be:
1. Maintaining the client's extremities in functional alignment
2. Encouraging the client to be out of bed to promote mobility
3. Supplying two or three pillows to place under painful joints
4. Performing range of motion every 2 hours to prevent contractures

258. The nurse does a discharge assessment of a newborn. A finding that would necessitate notifying the physician would be the presence of:
1. A round, protruding abdomen
2. Irregular, abdominal breathing
3. A liver palpable under the rib cage
4. Drainage at base of the umbilical cord

259. When reviewing discharge instructions with a client having preterm labor contractions, the nurse should instruct the client to:
1. Take the terbutaline only when she experiences contractions
2. Drink at least 8 to 10 (8 oz) cups of noncaffeinated fluids per day
3. Substitute other forms of sexual pleasure such as breast massage for intercourse
4. Try walking to see if she is having true labor contractions before notifying the physician

260. The nurse's dietary instructions will need to be modified when the pregnant adolescent says:
1. "You mean I don't have to give up my favorite foods like my mom says."
2. "Why do they want me to gain 35 pounds when a baby only weighs 7 pounds?"
3. "How am I ever going to lose all this weight they want me to gain while I'm pregnant?"
4. "I read in my magazine that the doctors don't care how much weight you gain any more."

261. When implementing a teaching plan focusing on self care for an autistic child, it is important for the nurse to:
1. Initially ask what the child would like to learn
2. Teach the child one aspect of the plan at a time
3. Include the child in group teaching with other children of the same age
4. Maintain close physical contact with the child while teaching, so that the child is better able to pay attention

262. When planning school interventions for a child with the diagnosis of attention deficit hyperactivity disorder, both the nurse and the teacher should remember to:
1. Provide as much structure as possible for the child
2. Tell the classmates that the child has trouble sitting still but is really trying
3. Encourage the mother to get the child into play therapy at a counselling center
4. Remove the child from the classroom when disruptive behavior is displayed to help the child gain some self control

263. A client is concerned about the development of tardive dyskinesia from phenothiazine use. The nurse should teach the client that:
    1. Although the symptoms are embarrassing, clients simply need to learn to live with them
    2. Although the symptoms are startling, they are not dangerous and respond readily to treatment
    3. The sleepiness, sedation, drooping of the eyelids, and strabismus will usually resolve spontaneously
    4. The chewing movements, restless legs, posturing of the head, and snakelike twistings occur only after prolonged use of the drug

264. During the first meeting of a therapy group one member of the group disagrees with any statement that is made by any other member. Because this is the first meeting of the group, the most therapeutic response by the nurse would be to:
    1. Point out the negative comments to this client and have the group explore the client's behavior
    2. Acknowledge the client's negative comments and ask the other clients to give feedback to the client
    3. Ignore this client's negative comments and encourage other members to continue to express their ideas
    4. Acknowledge the client's negative comments and attempt to find ways to help this client express positive comments

265. When reviewing the test results of a client scheduled for kidney surgery, the nurse should plan to notify the surgeon if it is noted that the:
    1. Hemoglobin is 10 g/dl and the hematocrit is 30%
    2. Urine contains a trace of protein and a trace of acetone
    3. Serum potassium is 3.7 mEq/L and the sodium is 140 mEq/L
    4. Serum creatinine is 1.6 mg/dl and the urea nitrogen is 28 mg/dl

266. Prior to giving preoperative care to a client scheduled for a coronary artery bypass graft, the nurse should be aware that:
    1. The client will need to retire from work following the surgery
    2. Surgery will always relieve the client's present anginal symptoms
    3. The basic mechanism causing atherosclerosis can be halted by this surgery
    4. The client has already undergone many related anxiety-provoking experiences

267. A client with a long history of IV drug abuse is in an accident and keeps asking for more pain medication. It would be most theraputic for the nurse to:
    1. Medicate the client if there is an order for analgesia and no contraindications
    2. Give the client something for pain orally instead of intramuscularly or intravenously
    3. Call the physician about this and have the physician develop a plan to treat the pain
    4. Get a physician's order for a nonsteroid antiinflammatory drug that may work without the problem of addiction

268. A client states to the nurse, "The doctor was bugging me about my blood pressure. I don't have high blood pressure. I don't have a blood pressure problem. I wish they'd leave me alone about my blood pressure." The nurse's best response would be:
    1. "Tell me, how high was it?"
    2. "Sounds like that really bothers you."
    3. "Let's talk about things you can do to bring it down."
    4. "You are upset because you have high blood pressure."

269. When questioned by a client with newly diagnosed insulin-dependent diabetes mellitus, the nurse explains that it is a chronic disease involving multiple body systems that results from:
    1. Alteration in glucose metabolism in the liver and large muscles
    2. Increased production of antidiabetic hormones from the pituitary gland
    3. Insufficient or absent enzyme formation by specialized alpha cells in the pancreas
    4. Decreased secretion or absence of the hormone produced in the beta cells of the pancreas

270. While taking the health history of a male client with uncontrolled insulin-dependent diabetes mellitus, the nurse learns that the client sometimes omits the prescribed daily insulin, "but always eats three meals a day." The diet prescribed is a 2200 calorie diabetic diet. The nurse recognizes that teaching for this client must include information on:

1. Ketoacidosis
   2. Lipodystrophy
   3. The symptoms of an insulin reaction
   4. Reducing intake when insulin is omitted

271. The physician has ordered 10 grains of aspirin every 4 hours for a client with rheumatoid arthritis. The pharmacy has supplied ASA 325 mg per tablet. Every 4 hours the nurse should administer:
   1. 1 tablet
   2. 2 tablets
   3. 1.5 tablets
   4. 2.5 tablets

272. While talking with the nurse about a problem with chronic constipation, the client describes a diet high in meats, dairy, breads, and diet sodas. The nurse's best response would be:
   1. "You've not been eating enough high fiber foods or drinking enough water."
   2. "You have not mentioned any fruits and vegetables; how often do you eat them?"
   3. "An occasional laxative will help you as long as you don't take them too frequently."
   4. "Sounds like you may develop a problem with cholesterol or gout; let's talk about the fat in your diet."

273. The physician prescribes an anticholinergic medication for an elderly client with Parkinson's disease. The nurse informs the client's family that a common side effect is:
   1. Dyskinesia
   2. Sleepiness
   3. Constipation
   4. Hypotension

274. A postpartal client confides to the nurse that she has heard that resumption of sexual relations can be painful and she wants to know why. The nurse explains that this can occur because of:
   1. Changes in the cervical os
   2. Increased maternal fatigue
   3. Alterations in vaginal rugae
   4. Decreased vaginal lubrication

275. Suspecting that a newborn has a congenital hip displacement, the nurse teaches the mother to put double diapers on the baby. This intervention is indicated by the nursing diagnosis of:
   1. High risk for injury
   2. Posttrauma response
   3. Altered tissue perfusion
   4. Altered patterns of urinary elimination

276. During an initial newborn assessment, the nurse discovers the newborn has a heart murmur. The nurse's next action should be to:
   1. Keep the infant NPO
   2. Notify the parents that the baby has a heart defect
   3. Take vital signs and blood pressures on all extremities
   4. Notify the infant's physician and prepare the infant for surgery

277. On the second day following open heart surgery, a 3-year-old toddler has a left chest tube connected to a water-seal drainage system. The nurse's assessment related to the chest tube should focus on:
   1. The patency of the chest tube
   2. When the chest tube system was changed
   3. Degree of bubbling of the chest tube system
   4. Amount of pain that the child is experiencing

278. A 26-year-old client has had pain in the right calf for 2 days. On examination the right calf is warm, red, edematous, and tender to touch. The nurse should ask the client if the pain is:
   1. Worse in the morning upon arising
   2. Increased with activity and alleviated with rest
   3. Relieved by placing the leg in a dependent position
   4. Aggravated when the toes are pointed toward the knee

279. A client with COPD also has hypertension. A classification of antihypertensive drugs that is contraindicated for clients with COPD is:
   1. Diuretics
   2. Vasodilators
   3. Beta-blocking agents
   4. ACE enzyme inhibitors

280. Kaposi's sarcoma often occurs in individuals with AIDS. The nurse is aware that Kaposi's sarcoma:
   1. Is rapidly progressive and infectious
   2. Causes brown discoloration of the feet
   3. Causes difficulty in walking and moving
   4. May invade internal organs and mucous membranes

281. A client's husband who has accompanied his wife to the labor room asks the nurse what "effaced" means. The nurse explains that this refers to the:
 1. Thinning of the cervical os
 2. Widening of the cervical os
 3. Rate of descent of the fetus
 4. Engorgement of cervical vessels

282. A client has an aortoiliac bypass and returns to the surgical unit with a nasogastric tube, Foley catheter, and IV fluids. On the first postoperative day, assessments related to this type of surgery about which the nurse should notify the surgeon immediately are:
 1. Urine output of 40 ml per hour, hemoglobin of 12.4 mg, abdominal pain
 2. A large diarrheal stool, absent right pedal pulse, urine output of 20 ml per hour
 3. Crackles in the lung bases, nasogastric drainage of 250 ml, weak pedal pulses
 4. Absence of bowel sounds, gastric drainage of 300 ml, white cell count of 11,000

283. When assessing a child with cerebral palsy, the nurse finds the child's ability to walk is impaired because of tendon deformities. The nurse identifies that the child walks:
 1. On the toes
 2. Pigeon-toed
 3. On the heels
 4. Knock-kneed

284. The nurse would expect that a pregnant woman who has tested positive for HIV/AIDS would respond by:
 1. Making an appointment to terminate the pregnancy
 2. Accepting the fact that the infant will be HIV-infected
 3. Accurately following the prescribed antiviral drug therapy plan
 4. Expecting the infant to show symptoms of the HIV infection immediately

285. A 17-year-old enters the emergency room complaining of sharp, low abdominal pain. She states her last normal period was 2 months ago. The nurse notes the client is pale and shaky. The client's vital signs are: B/P 86/42; T 99.8° F; P 132, thready and weak; R 32, and shallow. The nurse suspects an ectopic pregnancy. The nurse should first:
 1. Secure blood for a HIV titre
 2. Prepare the client for an amniocentesis
 3. Prepare the client for a pelvic examination
 4. Secure blood for an hCG, hemoglobin, and a hematocrit

286. A client receiving a tocolytic medication for control of preterm labor begins to experience tachycardia, hypotension, tremors, and a headache. The nurse recognizes these symptoms are probably related to the side effects of:
 1. Nifedipine
 2. Terbutaline
 3. Indomethacin
 4. Magnesium sulfate

287. Two weeks following delivery a client tells the nurse midwife that her nipples are sore and leaking a bloody, foul discharge. The nurse is aware that this:
 1. Occurs frequently in breastfeeding mothers
 2. Is indicative of mastitis in breastfeeding mothers
 3. Warrants an immediate mammogram to rule out malignancy
 4. Has resulted from too much pressure from the baby's mouth during nursing

288. A 45-year-old woman with a well differentiated, 1 cm, infiltrating breast cancer in the right breast is admitted for surgery. The admission assessment by the nurse should include a history of the breast mass and a:
 1. Family history of cancer, number of children, and any childbearing before 18 years of age
 2. Personal history of cancer, any symptoms of menopause, and mother's age at menopause
 3. Personal and family history of cancer; age at menarche, menopause, and at birth of first child; and number of children
 4. Personal and family history of cancer, age at menarche and menopause, number of children, and number of sex partners

289. An 18-year-old is admitted to the emergency room for a heroin overdose. The most dangerous symptom that the nurse would expect to see as a direct result of a heroin overdose is:
 1. Flushed face
 2. Dilated pupils
 3. Decreased respirations
 4. Increased blood pressure

290. The morning report indicates a client is agitated, angry, and frightened. The nurse validates this behavior, but time does not allow for a one-to-one interaction before the community meeting. It would be most therapeutic for the nurse to:
    1. Allow the client to temporarily withdraw from this activity
    2. Cajole the client into participating in the required community meeting
    3. Force the client to attend the community meeting to comply with the unit rules
    4. Give the prescribed prn medication and then persuade the client to attend the meeting with the nurse

291. A client with a long history of psychotic behavior, which has been controlled by antipsychotic drugs, is admitted with hyperpyrexia, muscle rigidity, altered mental status, and symptoms of autonomic instability. Neuroleptic malignant syndrome is diagnosed. The nursing diagnosis most appropriate in terms of priority for this client at this time would be:
    1. Hyperthermia
    2. Decreased cardiac output
    3. Impaired verbal communication
    4. Altered cardiopulmonary tissue perfusion

292. Preoperative teaching of a client who is to undergo a coronary bypass graft (CABG) should include the fact that:
    1. Ambulation will occur the evening of surgery
    2. An external cardiac pacemaker will be in place
    3. There will be an inability to swallow for several days
    4. A respirator will be used for the first week after surgery

293. Following arthroscopic surgery of the knee, a client is worried about the outcome because there are several incisions in the knee. To allay the client's fears, the nurse should explain that the:
    1. Incisions were made to allow for drainage following surgery
    2. Although multiple incisions cause pain, they do not affect the outcome
    3. Physician had to manipulate the knee in various ways during the procedure
    4. Multiple incisions were required to allow for adequate inspection of a variety of angles

294. A client has just returned from a cardiac catheterization. The nurse assesses the catheter site and notes profuse bleeding through the pressure dressing. The priority nursing action would be to:
    1. Elevate the affected extremity
    2. Notify the physician immediately
    3. Place pressure 1 inch above the catheter insertion site
    4. Change the dressing and apply a sterile 4 × 4 and pressure dressing

295. A lumbar puncture is ordered. The nurse is aware that during the procedure the client is positioned on the side to:
    1. Reduce the pain during the procedure
    2. Increase the space between the vertebrae
    3. Reduce the danger of damage to the spinal cord
    4. Decrease the chance of any respiratory complications

296. The nurse knows that health teaching has been effective when the mother of a child who was exposed to rabies from a raccoon bite states:
    1. "I'm so glad that these rabies shots kill the germ."
    2. "We'll come back four more times this month to get the rabies shots."
    3. "My daughter is getting the same rabies shots that dogs get every year."
    4. "I don't know how we will be able to catch the raccoon to see if it had rabies."

297. The nurse is able to evaluate that the parents understand their son's prescribed magnetic resonance imaging (MRI) test to detect a brain tumor when they state:
    1. "The test will take 5 minutes."
    2. "Our son has to take off his wireframe glasses."
    3. "His fillings might get pulled out by the machine."
    4. "Our son can't eat anything for 8 hours before the test."

298. A hospitalized 8-year-old is overheard in a crying toddler's room saying, "Be quiet. They'll hit you if you don't stop crying." The nurse would recognize that the nursing diagnosis with the highest priority for the 8-year-old would be:
   1. Fear related to hospitalization
   2. Risk for trauma related to suspected child abuse
   3. Altered thought processes related to developmental age
   4. Risk for violence directed toward the toddler related to verbal threat

299. The nurse should assess a child for plumbism by inquiring about:
   1. The intellegence level of all members of the family
   2. The family's past and current socioeconomic status
   3. The age of the home or apartment where the family resides
   4. The level of fluoride in the water supply in the school and home

300. A nurse asks a male client with a history of drug use, disturbed behavior, and loss of employment to write down a list of his strengths. The client states, "I don't have any strengths. How can you expect me to write anything? What should I do?" An appropriate nursing diagnosis at this time would be:
   1. Chronic low self-esteem related to the pain and humiliation of failure
   2. Impaired verbal communication related to feelings of anger and panic
   3. Social isolation related to feelings of distrust and inadequate feedback
   4. Altered thought processes related to inaccurate perceptions of self and others

Appendix A
State and Territorial Boards of Nursing

Alabama

Board of Nursing
RSA Plaza, Suite 250
770 Washington Avenue
Montgomery, Alabama 36130

Alaska

Board of Nursing
Department of Commerce & Economic Development
Division of Occupational Licensing
P.O. Box 110806
Juneau, Alaska 99811-0806

Arizona

Board of Nursing
1651 East Morten, Suite 150
Phoenix, Arizona 85020

Arkansas

Board of Nursing
University Tower Building, Suite 800
1123 S. University Avenue
Little Rock, Arkansas 72204

California

Board of Registered Nursing
P.O. Box 944210
400 R. Street, Suite 4030
Sacramento, California 95814-6200

Colorado

Board of Nursing
1560 Broadway, Suite 670
Denver, Colorado 80202

Connecticut

Board of Examiners for Nursing
150 Washington Street
Hartford, Connecticut 06106

Delaware

Board of Nursing
Cannon Building
P.O. Box 1401
861 Silver Lake Boulevard
Dover, Delaware 19903-1401

District of Columbia

Board of Nursing
614 H. Street NW
Washington, D.C. 20001

Florida

Board of Nursing
111 E. Coastline Drive, Suite 516
Jacksonville, Florida 32202

Georgia

Board of Nursing
166 Pryor Street SW, Suite 400
Atlanta, Georgia 30303

Guam

Board of Nurse Examiners
Box 2816
Agana, Guam 96910

Hawaii

Board of Nursing
Box 3469
Honolulu, Hawaii 96801

Idaho

Board of Nursing
P.O. Box 83720
2800 N. 8th Street, Suite 210
Boise, Idaho 83720-0061

Illinois
Department of Professional Regulation
320 W. Washington Street, 3rd Floor
Springfield, Illinois 62786

Indiana
State Board of Nursing
Health Professions Bureau
402 W. Washington Street, Room 041
Indianapolis, Indiana 46204

Iowa
Board of Nursing
1223 E. Court
Des Moines, Iowa 50319

Kansas
State Board of Nursing
Landon State Office Bldg.
900 SW Jackson, Room 551-S
Topeka, Kansas 66612-1230

Kentucky
Board of Nursing
312 Whittington Parkway, Suite 300
Louisville, Kentucky 40222-5172

Louisiana
Board of Nursing
150 Baronne Street, Room 912
New Orleans, Louisiana 70112

Maine
Board of Nursing
35 Anthony Avenue
State House Station 158
Augusta, Maine 04333

Maryland
Board of Nursing
4140 Patterson Avenue
Baltimore, Maryland 21215-2254

Massachusetts
Board of Registration in Nursing
Government Center
100 Cambridge Street, Room 1519
Boston, Massachusetts 02202

Michigan
Board of Nursing
P.O. Box 30018
Lansing, Michigan 48909

Minnesota
Board of Nursing
2700 University Avenue W, Suite 108
St. Paul, Minnesota 55114

Mississippi
Board of Nursing
239 N. Lamar Street, Suite 401
Jackson, Mississippi 39201

Missouri
Board of Nursing
3605 Missouri Blvd.
P.O. Box 656
Jefferson City, Missouri 65102

Montana
Board of Nursing
Department of Commerce
P.O. Box 200513
111 N. Jackson
Helena, Montana 59620-0513

Nebraska
Board of Nursing
P.O. Box 95007
Lincoln, Nebraska 68509

Nevada
Board of Nursing
1281 Terminal Way, Suite 116
Reno, Nevada 89502

New Hampshire
Board of Nursing
Division of Public Health Services
Health & Welfare Building
6 Hazen Drive
Concord, New Hampshire 03301

New Jersey
Board of Nursing
124 Halsey Street
Newark, New Jersey 07102

New Mexico
Board of Nursing
4206 Louisiana Boulevard NE
Albuquerque, New Mexico 87109-1807

New York

Board of Nursing
New York State Education Department, Room 3023
Cultural Education Center
Albany, New York 12230

North Carolina

Board of Nursing
P.O. Box 2129
Raleigh, North Carolina 27602-2129

North Dakota

Board of Nursing
919 S. 7th Street, Suite 504
Bismarck, North Dakota 58504-5881

Ohio

Board of Nursing
77 S. High Street, 17th Floor
Columbus, Ohio 43266-0316

Oklahoma

Board of Nursing
2915 N. Classen Boulevard, Suite 524
Oklahoma City, Oklahoma 73106

Oregon

Board of Nursing
800 NE Oregon Street, Suite 465
Portland, Oregon 97232

Pennsylvania

Board of Nursing
P.O. Box 2649
Harrisburg, Pennsylvania 17105-2649

Puerto Rico

Board of Nurse Examiners
Call Box 10200
Santurce, Puerto Rico 00908-0200

Rhode Island

Board of Nursing Registration and Education
Cannon Health Building, Room 104
3 Capitol Hill
Providence, Rhode Island 02908-5097

South Carolina

Board of Nursing
Winthrop Building
220 Executive Center Drive, Suite 220
Columbia, South Carolina 29210-8422

South Dakota

Board of Nursing
3307 S. Lincoln Avenue
Sioux Falls, South Dakota 57105

Tennessee

Board of Nursing
Bureau of Manpower and Facilities
283 Plus Park Boulevard.
Nashville, Tennessee 37247-1010

Texas

Board of Nurse Examiners
9101 Burnet Road, Suite 104
Austin, Texas 78758

Utah

Board of Nursing
Heber M. Wells Building, 4th Floor
160 E. 300 South
PO Box 45805
Salt Lake City, Utah 84145-0805

Vermont

Board of Nursing
109 State Street
Montpelier, Vermont 05609-1106

Virgin Islands

Board of Nurse Licensure
Kongens Gade #3
P.O. Box 4247
St. Thomas, Virgin Islands 00803

Virginia

Board of Nursing
6606 West Broad Street, 4th Floor
Richmond, Virginia 23230

Washington

Washington State Nursing Care
Quality Assurance Commission
P.O. Box 47864
Olympia, Washington 98504-7864

West Virginia

Board of Examiners for RNs
101 Dee Drive
Charleston, West Virginia 25311

Wisconsin

Board of Nursing
1400 E. Washington Avenue, Room 174
P.O. Box 8935
Madison, Wisconsin 53708-8935

Wyoming

Board of Nursing
Barrett Bldg., 2nd Floor
2301 Central Avenue
Cheyenne, Wyoming 82002

Appendix B
Canadian Provincial Registered Nurses Associations

Alberta

Alberta Association of Registered Nurses
11620 168th Street
Edmonton, Alberta
T5M 4A6
(403) 451-0043

British Columbia

Registered Nurses Association of British Columbia
2855 Arbutus Street
Vancouver, British Columbia
V6Y 3Y8
(604) 736-7731

Manitoba

Manitoba Association of Registered Nurses
647 Broadway Avenue
Winnipeg, Manitoba
R3C 0X2
(204) 774-3477

New Brunswick

Nurses Association of New Brunswick
231 Saunders Street
Fredericton, New Brunswick
E3B 1N6
(506) 458-8731

Newfoundland

Association of Registered Nurses of Newfoundland
55 Military Road
P.O. Box 6116
St. John's, Newfoundland
A1C 5X8
(709) 753-6040

Northwest Territories

Northwest Territories Registered Nurses Association
P.O. Box 2757
Yellowknife, Northwest Territories
X1A 2R1
(403) 873-2745

Nova Scotia

Registered Nurses Association of Nova Scotia
6035 Coburg Road
Halifax, Nova Scotia
B3H 1Y8
(902) 423-6156

Ontario

College of Nurses of Ontario
101 Davenport Road
Toronto, Ontario
M5R 3PI
(416) 928-0900

Prince Edward Island

Association of Nurses of Prince Edward Island
PO Box 1838
Charlottetown, Prince Edward Island
C1A 7N5
(902) 892-6322

Quebec

Ordre des infirmieres et infirmiers du Quebec
4200 Quest, Boulevard Dorchester
Montreal, Quebec
H3Z 1V4
(514) 935-2501

Saskatchewan

Saskatchewan Registered Nurses Association
2066 Retallack Street
Regina, Saskatchewan
S4T 2K2
(306) 757-4643

Yukon

Yukon Nurses Society
P.O. Box 5371
Whitehorse, Yukon
Y1A 4Z2
(403) 667-4062